DIET FOR GREAT SEX

Food for Male and Female
Sexual Health

Christine DeLozier, L.Ac.

Cover and interior illustration design by Morgan Wittmer
Logo Meg Spoto, mdashstudio.com
Cover images by photomaru, Morgan Wittmer
Edited by Tracy Moore
Recipes images by Emily Daniels, Artjazz, Elena Veselova, Olga Lepeshkina, Marian Vejcik, Natalia Lisovskaya, Evgeny Labutin
Interior design by Amie McCracken

This book is dedicated to my sister, Cori
What would I do without you?

TABLE OF CONTENTS

Introduction...9

Part I: The Science of a Great Sex Diet.................................13

Hormones

Hormonal Balance and Great Sex......................................14
Eating to Balance Hormones...21

Nerves

The Nervous System and Great Sex...................................37
Mushrooms, Nerves and Great Sex....................................47

Blood

The Vascular System and Great Sex...................................57
Minerals..69

Part II: Ancient Chinese Wisdom for Great Sex................79
Traditional Chinese Medicine Past and Present 80
Traditional Chinese Dietetics for Great Sex 89

Part III: Environment and Lifestyle for Great Sex............99
Great Sex is in the Living and Breathing........................100
Heavy Metal Exposure..106
Electromagnetic Fields..113
Great Sex from Your Partner's Eyes 119
Aphrodisiacs: Fluffers of the Gods 133

Part IV: The Fun Part: Practicing What You've Learned....159
Great Sex Action Plan 160
Bonus: A Few Tips to Give You Some Game in the Bedroom...........198

Acknowledgements...221
About the Author...223
References by Chapter...225

INTRODUCTION

Hot sex. *Naturally.* That's what this book is about. We all want to have it, but the pathway can be more elusive than we might imagine. It's what drives so many people to my acupuncture practice, where I help individuals and couples to have better sex. Men come in seeking stronger erections. Women come looking to improve libido and sexual satisfaction. Why do they come to me for help?

Acupuncture moves qi in the vessels, stimulating nerve pathways which affect every substance produced by the body, including sex hormones. It also brings blood flow to the sex organs, which is essential for male and female sexual function.

The philosophy of traditional Chinese medicine is to always address the *root* of health concerns. The root of sexual function involves our diet. We are born with yin and yang in perfect balance, but our lifestyles can block qi and blood from flowing to our sex organs.

But what *should* humans eat? This has long been a scientific debate with experts voicing strong opinions. Other primates seem to inherently know what foods promote health, while humans rely on nutrition experts to tell us what to eat. I saw a documentary about monkeys who lived in Indian cities, hanging out on rooftops. They would go around stealing food from vendors and from people's houses. Since we have lost our natural inclinations for what food is good for us, I am always curious to see what our biological cousins like to eat.

These monkeys would sneak in open windows and emerge with whole squash. They staked out farm stands and swooped in to steal fresh mangos and other ripe fruit. In my private practice I was seeing patients every day whose diets were wreaking havoc on their sex lives. I decided to take a scientific look at which foods naturally support great sex.

The fruits of that research fill *Diet for Great Sex: Food for Male and Female Sexual Health*. Long before I became interested in acupuncture, I trained to become a research scientist. Drawing on that training, I have spent countless hours reviewing clinical and epidemiological research in writing this book. The chapters are filled with the wide range of evidence that prove in modern scientific terms the dietary path to great sex.

Physiologically, great sex is achieved by balanced sex hormones, fast nerve impulses to and from the genitals and blood vessels which deliver optimal blood flow. Modern research proves that diet affects this trifecta of great sex and can increase or hamper pleasure.

Hormones. Nerve pathways. Blood flow.

We must care for the biological design of our bodies. A great deal of clinical research demonstrates that certain eating habits increase blood flow to the genitals, balance sex hormones and help nerves to be most responsive to our partner's touch.

Diet affects sex. For example, did you know that leafy greens contain nutrients which reduce cortisol and normalize testosterone? We have the science to prove it. They also improve the elasticity of blood vessels and increase nitric oxide, which bring more blood flow to the genitals. Fatty, salty foods, on the other hand, stiffen blood vessels in a matter of hours, leading to reduced blood flow. Did you also know that blood flow is not important only for males? It's also essential for female pleasure and orgasm.

What we take into our bodies must nurture the essences of sex. With yin and yang in harmony, we can bring out all that is possible from our own sensual physiology.

In *Diet for Great Sex*, you'll find an entire chapter on the role of sex hormones, which need proper balance to regulate everything from arousal, libido, and orgasm, to stress, sleep habits, and general well-being.

I'll cover the function of the nervous system, and qi, as it relates to sexual health. Proper nerve conduction is essential to great sex, and we'll talk about what dietary habits and nutrients we need to help nerves fire strong signals to and from the sex organs.

You'll meet your vascular system, which delivers qi and blood to our genitals for great sex. You'll learn which foods to eat and avoid to increase blood flow and remove blockage. It takes surprisingly little time to see improvements.

I'll explain traditional Chinese dietary therapy, and we'll discuss the meridians, or vessels, that carry qi and blood throughout the body and how to ensure free flow. Quite often, you'll see, traditional Chinese medicine and modern science merge on many key aspects of great sexual function.

While this book is a guide to eating well for incredible sex, it also explores culinary aphrodisiacs. These aphrodisiacs (real and mythologized) can be incorporated into your diet for enhancing libido, and I'll clear up some longstanding misconceptions (ahem, Spanish Fly). Saffron and nutmeg, for example, are safe and have actually been scientifically studied for their benefit to sexual function.

Diet for Great Sex also addresses some of the environmental threats to our sexual health, as well as the mind-body balance. Helping our bodies achieve their best rhythms are exercise and better sleep. You'll also find practical advice for achieving greater harmony through mutual respect and kindness as lovers. In addition, detailed tips for pleasing your partner are provided.

Finally, everything comes together in a great sex action plan with delicious recipes. The book contains meal plans, sample menus and a dietary planner. Also included is a date-night sex menu for a night of passion and better blood flow.

Who should read *Diet for Great Sex*? Anyone who would like to have the best sex possible, through the most natural means possible. This includes people who already have great sex and want to keep it that way, as well as those who want it to be better.

This book uses scientific evidence to uncover the best dietary habits for great sex, merging modern science with traditional Chinese medicine, a centuries-long guide to better sexual function. In a body that is well cared for, where qi and blood move freely, desire comes to us naturally, pleasure comes to us naturally, and orgasm is effortless.

PART I:
THE SCIENCE OF
A GREAT SEX DIET

HORMONAL BALANCE AND GREAT SEX

It was their third date. Based on the steamy texts and innuendo they'd shared for weeks, Carla and Dan knew that sex was in the cards tonight. But as they flirted their way through chicken alfredo and crème brûlée, they both began feeling a bit nervous about the main event. After all, it would be their first time exploring their sexual compatibility, and that was always a gamble. They arrived at his place and headed straight for the bedroom, falling into the sheets. Their desire and enthusiasm led the way, but as they undressed, something else took over.

Immediately, Dan couldn't help wondering what Carla was thinking as she gazed at his body. *It would be easier for her to see my dick if my gut weren't in the way,* he thought, suddenly hearing a lifetime-long chorus of dick jokes materialize in his head. *Does she think I'm inadequate? I'm sure her other boyfriends were packing way more heat.* Suddenly he noticed his sheets smelled rank and hoped she didn't notice too. He moved to start caressing Carla's naked body, making his way down between her legs.

As for Carla, she really liked Dan, and hoped he liked her just as much. She wanted the sex to be perfect, but as his hands made their way down south, she became increasingly self-conscious about what he was thinking.

Carla, suddenly conjuring a highlight reel of perfect porn-star genitalia snapshots in her mind's eye, imagined Dan would discover she was less waxed, bleached and youthfully sculpted down there and more like a finely aged USDA beef—dry aged. The juices weren't flowing on command. She knew climax for her was far more likely with a long-term boyfriend, as it is for many heterosexual women, but she would've been more than good with successful penetration. *He probably thinks I'm not into sex. Frigid. That's just what turns a guy on, a woman who can't get off.* Her libido had always been on the low side, too, which had led to a lot of frustrated partners in previous relationships.

Thanks to the wine with dinner, they did finally make it to sex, doggie style. Here, Dan felt a bit awkward again. What to do with his hands? Should he grab her hips? Ass? Put them on his own hips? Go slow? Try a bit of roughness? He caught a glimpse in the mirror of his gut slapping against her ass and cringed. His erection began to soften.

This was a new development. When he was twenty, his erections had been like concrete at the mere hint of sex, but now he had to work at it a bit more, and at a recent check-up, his doctor said that his testosterone was low.

Dan and Carla were certainly experiencing first-time sex jitters, always a possibility between new partners. But as an acupuncturist and herbalist, I saw something else lurking in those sheets: hormonal imbalance, which was affecting their game in bed. Their dinner — fatty, salty and rich— was just the sort of food that was working against their efforts at pleasure. Because diet affects hormonal balance, nerve integrity and vascular health—the holy trinity of great sex. And a crappy diet will hamper the physiology of great sex faster than Dan can grab a cold shower or Carla can hope her vibrator batteries still have life left in them.

***

I treat patients like Dan and Carla in my acupuncture practice, where I work with clients individually and as couples to cultivate healthy nerves, healthy blood vessels and hormonal balance. I treat patients with acupuncture but always combine this with an individualized dietary strategy to support sexual function as this is the single best way to maintain sexual health.

Acupuncture, an ancient Chinese form of healing therapy, operates on the nervous system, stimulating nerve pathways to improve sexual function. The nervous system in turn, affects the levels of every substance produced by the body. Science has shown that acupuncture affects a broad range of chemical messengers from dopamine, norepinephrine and the fight-or-flight hormone cortisol, to histamine, a compound critical in immune response. Sexually speaking, acupuncture has also been found to affect both free and total testosterone in the body,[1] as well as estradiol, a form of estrogen, both of which are key players in our sexual function.[2]

Medical jargon aside, though, the takeaway is simple: Hormones affect sex, and diet affects hormones. Certain dietary habits improve hormonal balance, while others derail it mercilessly.

So even when you address the insecurity, unfamiliarity, lack of skill or good old-fashioned nervousness that plagues us all from time to time in the bedroom, hormones and diet are two critical elements of sexual function. When ignored, they can make for bad sex. But tame them both and you unlock the key to sexual satisfaction. (Though you'll still have to wash your sheets.)

First, the hormones.

Hormones and Sex

The endocrine system is our chemical communications system that produces hormones or messengers in the body. Think of them as the messengers who shape the very narrative of our well-being, controlling our blood sugar, our energy levels, our stress response, our sleep schedule and even our fertility. They are the town criers of our bodies, telling us when we are hungry, when we are full, when we are sleepy and, most importantly to my clients like Carla and Dan, when we are horny.

They are key players in sexual function. Arousal? It all depends on hormones such as testosterone and estrogen, among numerous others. Libido? Hormones. Erections? Hormones. Lubrication? Hormones. Pleasure? Say it with me: hormones!

While it isn't essential for the layperson to grasp every hormone's complex function in the body or the bedroom in order to gain a little mastery over them, what's important to grasp here is how critical they are to great sex, and how much control we really do have in aiding them in their goals.

Ancient Chinese medicine awoke to this reality long before Western medicine took notice, observing hormonal balance as the continual interaction between yin and yang. Yin and yang are the way of heaven and earth, through which one can understand all phenomena in the universe, including sex. Yin is the cool, feminine dampness of a winter night. It is the earth. Yang is the hot, masculine scorching of a summer day. It is the heavens. Heaven and earth became disconnected in us, but in sex, yin and yang essences merge once again between us and within us.

Please note that even though I'm using feminine and masculine here in line with the way traditional Chinese medicine (TCM) does, we all contain yin and yang within each of us. For this reason, Chinese medicine also has a unique advantage in treating and aiding everyone, including the gender fluid, because it focuses on how these elements differ in the individual and can be calibrated within us, no matter our identity or orientation. (For the sake of presenting medical research, I'll use the terms "male and female bodies" to refer to subjects' born biological status. This is important in understanding the working force of hormones within the body on the biomedical level, which, again, can be calibrated based on the individual.)

The continual interaction between yin and yang can also be observed via modern science through the complex interplay of hormones. We see it in the monthly temperature changes that accompany menstruation, which cycle through a cool yin phase at the month's outset, culminating during ovulation, where yin transforms to hot yang, bringing basal body temperatures higher for the remainder of the month. In medical terms, estrogens and androgens also dance to enhance sexual arousal, peaking at ovulation and at the follicular phase of the menstrual cycle.

Hormonal balance is undoubtedly connected with great sex. For example, optimal testosterone means stronger erections in males and easier, more satisfying orgasms in females. Scientific research now helps us understand how we can enhance this relationship for increased sexual satisfaction. For instance, we can naturally optimize testosterone levels through diet, weight training, walking and other activities, as I'll discuss later in this book.

Testosterone is produced by the testes, the ovaries and also by the adrenal glands, which sit right on top of the kidneys. In TCM, the kidneys are understood to be the root of the essence, with male essence being sperm and female essence being menses. The kidneys, then, are thought to be at the center of sexual and reproductive health.

Males *generally* have higher testosterone than females. This is a very important physiological difference, as it affects a number of sexual features including libido. However, often misunderstood is that estrogen is also very important in males, who have an enzyme, aromatase, which converts testosterone to estradiol, a form of estrogen. Again, optimal estrogen is *also* associated in males with better and more sex, higher libido, improved ejaculation and orgasm and more night-time erections. This is because estrogen is needed to trigger the pituitary gland to release gonadotropins—hormones that stimulate the activity of the testes. It is also a major player in male fertility.

That said, optimal levels of androgens and estrogens are different for males and females. In relation to great sex, males do better with higher androgen levels and lower estrogen levels, while for females it is the opposite.

Of note, there is a difference between total testosterone and free testosterone. Most testosterone in the bloodstream is bound to a protein called sex-hormone binding globulin (SHBG). The remaining 2% is free and available for our bodies to use.

Adequate free testosterone is important because it improves memory, mathematical reasoning and cognitive ability. It also increases muscle mass. Low androgen levels increase risk of cardiovascular disease and insulin resistance. Improved testosterone levels can increase one's sense of well-being. Males with low free testosterone commonly complain of loss of libido, dysphoria (a state of unease and dissatisfaction with life), fatigue, irritability and depression. They also deal with weaker erections. These symptoms overlap with signs and symptoms of major depression. There is a significant inverse correlation between bioavailable testosterone and depression score in elderly males.

Both testosterone and estradiol have been shown to be important for female sexual desire. In females, estrogen supplementation typically increases libido, with a two-day lag, while progesterone consistently reduces it. However, in normal human levels, progesterone facilitates female sexual behavior.

Progesterone therapy has been used to control libido in felony sex offenders. However, in typical levels present in the body, it actually enhances masculine sexuality, stimulating sex behaviors.

Growth hormone and prolactin are not sex hormones per se, but they play a role in everyone's sexual function. Prolactin is a hormone associated with milk production in females but is also produced by males. Levels increase following orgasm in everyone and may affect subsequent arousal. Prolactin is also believed to exert influence on erectile strength, and genital sexual response. High prolactin is associated with hypogonadism and lower arousal across the board.

Low prolactin levels are associated with reduced erectile function, sexual satisfaction, and reduced quality of orgasm in males. In females, elevated prolactin levels were associated with depressive symptoms and reduced sexual desire, arousal, lubrication, orgasm and sexual satisfaction.[3]

As males age, and body fat increases, testosterone and DHEA (dehydroepiandrosterone) levels fall, while LH (luteinizing hormone), FSH (follicle-stimulating hormone) and SHBG (sex hormone-binding globulin) levels increase.[4] Smoking, age and obesity all affect sex hormones. Cigarette smokers have higher levels of DHEA, DHEAS and cortisol levels which, when in abundance, can wreak havoc. Alcohol consumption also increases cortisol levels to negative affect.

Diabetes, Insulin and Sex

A bit more about the effect of diabetes on our sexual function: Humans knew thousands of years ago that having diabetes caused ineptitude in the bedroom. Medieval Persian writer Avicenna wrote about diabetes in *The Canon of Medicine* (c.1025), describing "abnormal appetite, the collapse of sexual functions and the sweet taste of diabetic urine." Insulin is a hormone which allows our cells to utilize sugar, but, in the case of diabetes, the body is either resistant to it (Type 2 diabetes) or doesn't produce it (Type 1).

Wasting and Thirsting Disorder, as diabetes is called in TCM, is understood as an extremely deficient or blocked yin. Adequate yin substance is essential to fill the vessels of sexuality. For the numerous people with diabetes, this problem of yin causes sexual complaints. Diabetic patients have lower levels of sexual desire, sexual arousal, have sex less and less sexual satisfaction. Diabetics also have higher risk of erectile dysfunction. Those with the worst control over blood glucose levels have the most severe problems.[5]

One of the reasons diabetes affects sexual function is due to its damage of blood vessels, including those leading to the penis, clitoris and vagina.

Diabetes and insulin resistance interferes with both nitric oxide and testosterone production.[6] Blood flow is essential for pleasure and function in all of us. To make things worse, diabetes injures nerves. As diabetic damage occurs, nerves leading to and from the genitals lose their ability to send those crucial signals of pleasure and arousal. This, too, has a remedy: Diet can drastically improve Type 2 diabetes and its sexual side effects.

Serotonin and Dopamine

There are a few additional, critical chemical messengers involved in our sexual health. Serotonin is a neurohormone produced by our bodies which helps us to feel a sense of well-being. When injected in certain parts of the brain, serotonin will delay ejaculation, while in other parts of the brain, it will cause ejaculation to occur. In general though, increased serotonin will prolong the time between erection and ejaculation, which is why it is sometimes used as a treatment for premature ejaculation.

The pharmaceutical class of antidepressants, selective serotonin reuptake inhibitors (SSRI's) increase the availability of serotonin to improve mood. For this reason, SSRI's have sexual side-effects. Like serotonin, dopamine stimulation can cause ejaculation to occur, and certain classes of drugs that block certain dopamine receptors make ejaculation difficult or impossible. Other types of dopamine interference can cause premature ejaculation.

The level of one hormone influences levels of other hormones, so when they are out of balance, this can have a global effect on the body and hence, our sexuality. Hormones are rarely out of balance in isolation. For example, when we see unbalanced testosterone, we usually see unbalanced DHEA, estradiol, and vitamin D, among others, which is part of something called multiple hormonal dysregulation.

These hormones and chemical components should be acknowledged, tended to and fed well, and there is scientific research to show us how to do this effectively. In turn, with yin and yang in balance, sex, my friend, is a heavenly delight.

EATING TO
BALANCE HORMONES

Humans make everything so freaking complicated. Other animals, who are natural Casanovas, also possess the simple knowledge of what foods they should eat and take them just as they are from the hand of mother nature. Deer nibble berries from a bush. Squirrels gather nuts. Dogs catch a rabbit and eat it right there, bones and all.

Humans, on the other hand, decide a year in advance that wheat will be eaten. They plant the wheat. They water the wheat. They mill the wheat, and take out the fibrous exterior, grinding it into a fine powder. They mix the wheat with bird eggs, secretions from a lactating cow, fungus powder, powdered metal and dried cane sap from a plant that grows 3,000 miles away. They then heat all of these disassembled plant, animal, fungal and mineral parts until they congeal into what we call cake. Then they finally eat that wheat.

Simple things aren't good enough for us. We wouldn't eat corn right from the field. We'd rather boil the corn, stick the corn in a can and put it on a shelf for two years. Then only when we're good and ready, we boil that corn again and eat it. In fact, we can't be bothered to even get up and get the corn ourselves, preferring to make it a game of intrigue where we hire somebody to hide from the feds, sneak in and get the corn for us. Deer nibble corn from the stalk. Simple.

Humans, not innately knowing which plants and animals are good for us, rely on others to tell us what to eat. And as human nutrition experts, we don't seem to know what the hell we're talking about. We cut carbs, and increase fat, then we eat lots of carbs and no fat. We eat meat for iron and vitamin B-12, and then don't eat meat because it's too fatty.

Our hormones, nerves and blood vessels are the holy trinity of great sex. In order to find symphonic harmony, we need to feed them properly. For this reason, I interview my clients about what they eat in a given day.

Take Dan. He usually ate a truck driver's breakfast on the way to work every day—whatever he could grab from a gas station. Typically this was a huge donut with a green soda and a granola bar for a snack. He often had a working lunch with colleagues at a restaurant chosen for convenience, and he pulled his processed dinner directly out of the freezer to nuke.

Carla wasn't feeding her sexual appetite much better, munching on frequent baked goods from the coffee shop and iced-coffee smoothies loaded with sugary extras. Her busy professional job made cooking difficult, so she often ate pre-packaged meals like cheese and crackers with a cookie and juice box.

By now we've all heard relentlessly that the standard American diet (SAD) of high sugar, fat and processed foods is bad for us, but we haven't effectively broadcasted one of the worst byproducts of that diet: bad sex. The SAD diet makes for sad sex because it disrupts our sex hormones. Add to this that Americans are dealing the highest ever rates of Type 2 diabetes, which damages blood vessels and nerves, both critical to blood flow and sensation, impairing sexual pleasure and function.

All this played out behind the scenes during Carla and Dan's romantic encounter. Their high-sugar, high-fat diet was wreaking havoc on their hormonal balance, disruptions which likely affected a whole series of hormones, not just one. This meant a weak erection for Dan and left Carla high, dry and unsatisfied.

This is fixable. Simple dietary changes can move our sexual and endocrine health in the right direction. A diet for great sex hormones involves eating lower-fat while getting adequate vitamin D, fiber, B vitamins and leafy greens, all of which promote sexual endocrine balance and therefore better sexual function. It means adding in cruciferous vegetables, such as cauliflower and broccoli, which contain various phytonutrients that promote sexual health. It means implementing brief periods of fasting, which research has shown to help normalize hormones, and we'll talk about the best way to approach this.

Not-so-Sweet Spot: Refined Sugars and Hormonal Balance

Because refined sugar is a cheap, shelf-stable substance, soft drinks, fruit-flavored drinks and sweet bakery products are now the primary food sources of fructose in our diets, and they aren't doing us any favors with our love life. A high-fructose diet causes inflammation, oxidative stress as well as mitochondrial damage, and leads to obesity and metabolic syndrome.[7]

Traditional Chinese dietitians advise balancing all of the five flavors of sweet, sour, bitter, acrid and salty in the diet. These are flavors occurring in nature without the addition of table salt and sugar. For example, meat is salty, fruit is both sweet and sour, greens are bitter, garlic and ginger are acrid. The addition of so much added sugar in the diet disturbs this balance, causing disharmony of yin and yang, and disease ensues.

Disproportion of the five flavors upsets hormones. Favoring the sweet flavor over others, for example, disrupts leptin. Leptin is a hormone that is produced to tell us when we are full, inhibiting hunger. People at an unhealthy weight tend to be leptin resistant, which means that their bodies don't tell them that they are full when they should, so they end up taking in too many calories.[8] Refined sugars have been shown in research to induce leptin resistance.

Leptin also induces the synthesis of nitric oxide which assists erections and helps relax clitoral smooth muscles. This means that more blood flows to the clitoris for increased sexual pleasure and sexual response.

Here's a mouthful: Melanocortinergic agents. In the body these substantially improve hepatic (liver) insulin sensitivity, regulate energy expenditure and powerfully induce sexual arousal. For this reason, their role in erectile dysfunction is under investigation. In research, leptin resistance and insulin resistance lead to reduced melanocortin (MC) activity and impaired sexual function.[9]

High-fructose consumption causes alterations in dopamine pathways in the brain, which can compromise our sleep/wake cycles[10] and affect sexual function. A high-fat, high-sugar diet also negatively affects the reproduction cycle. In females, drinking more than one cup of sweetened soda per day is associated with significantly altered estradiol levels.[11]

Drinking sugar-sweetened beverages also lowers semen quality in males and reduces fertility in everyone.[12] Sugar-sweetened beverages are significantly associated with low serum testosterone in males.[13] One study found that high-fructose corn syrup reduces sperm count, testicular weight, testosterone levels and leads to pathological testicular tissue changes.[14]

So, you can see why Dan's high intake of sugar was likely contributing to his low testosterone and loss of erections. And since refined sugars interfere with estradiol levels, Carla's body was also not launching an adequate biological response to sexual stimulation. Though she wanted to have sex, her body did not produce lubricants when Dan touched and caressed her. It also indicates that blood did not engorge her vagina and clitoris, since this precedes lubrication. This engorgement is a major factor in female sexual pleasure and satisfaction.

Balancing Hormones

Here I'll outline how we can eat our way to hot, horny sex with some of the key vitamins, minerals and foods that give us the best shot at hormonal balance, and therefore sexual well-being.

Salad Tossing: Lessons from Other Primates

Humans are primates, just like chimpanzees and monkeys, but at some point in our evolution we lost the ability to instinctively eat what would most nourish health and thereby also nourish great sex. Many fad diets have tried to take a page from our primate cousins as to what mother nature intended for us to eat. The conclusions though have led to some pretty extreme dietary recommendations.

What we do know is that primates generally eat loads of vegetation. In fact, a huge portion of virtually all primates' diets contain copious amounts of leaves, fruit and often a much smaller amount of animal protein, usually bugs. With so much fruit and leaves, they take in many many times the quantities of essential minerals such as calcium, magnesium, zinc and potassium as modern humans.

As unsexy as it might sound, leaves are probably the single best thing you can put in your body for great sex (I do mean *eat*, but no judgment for other uses, so long as you're safe). They facilitate that holy trinity of great sex: hormonal balance, nerve integrity and vascular health. This one single vegetable is a triple hitter for sexual health.

In TCM, leafy greens are considered to be bitter in flavor, which is poorly represented in our modern diet. Instead we tend to favor sweet and salty flavors, which leads to imbalance.

Leafy greens restore balance to hormones affecting sex, such as cortisol, which is induced by stress and is a major libido-killer. Cortisol lowers testosterone levels, which, remember, is important for all of us. Females with high cortisol levels have more difficulty achieving orgasm and lower libido. And high cortisol for males affects sex at all levels. Leafy greens, which are rich in zinc, lower cortisol and improve testosterone levels to raise libido.

Thylakoids are found in the membranes of green leaves like romaine and green leaf lettuces. Thylakoids contain vitamins E and K, and anti-oxidants, like chlorophyll, which protect humans against disease. They act as a prebiotic, positively affecting gut flora and triggering the release of gut hormones, such as leptin, that tell us we are full and improve insulin sensitivity. Lactobacillus reuteri is an anti-obesity bacteria in the gut and significantly increased with thylakoids.[15]

Thylakoids suppress ghrelin and CCK, which are hunger signals, in response to both fatty and carbohydrate-rich meals. They also reduce blood lipids and blood glucose, which can generate inflammation. Thylakoids also help regulate blood sugar. Better yet, research shows that subjects given thylakoids showed decreased desire for sweets and fatty foods, both in the short term and in the long term, meaning it actively helps you curb cravings.

Natural nitrate-rich leafy greens also boost nitric oxide in the body. This improves the elasticity of blood vessels, for enhanced vascular health and increased blood flow to the genitals. We will discuss this more later.

Leafy greens are loaded with vital minerals and antioxidants, which have been shown in research to improve the speed and strength of nerve signals. This means that nerve impulses to and from our genitals are more robust, which directly equates to more sensitivity and more pleasure. It's no wonder that other primates spend such a great portion of their time eating leaves and getting it on.

Meat and Fiber

Ingestion of animal product in the diet of primates ranges from 0% in some species to more than 90% in others. Where humans fall in this range is a matter of debate.

Many primates that were once considered herbivores are now known to eat quite significant quantities of animal products when they are able to. They will intentionally eat more animal protein when it is economically possible. For example, in one study of baboons, an outbreak of grasshoppers led the baboons to shift their diet to almost entirely animal product. They changed their daily habits until the grasshopper outbreak was finished. Also, chimpanzees have been known to hunt baboons, and baboons have been known to hunt infant gazelles. While animal protein is often a small portion of their diet, it can be a significant one for sex.

For example, in many zoos, slow lorises are fed a diet of fruit and leaves, neglecting insects. In the wild, though, about 30% of their calories come from eating insects, birds and small reptiles. When lorises who were previously fed only plants were provided a cricket dispenser, their sexual behaviors increased.[16] So, with a diet which more closely corresponds to nature, sexual behaviors are normalized.

However, this does not mean that we should disregard all of the research showing that our high fat, high meat diets are causing disease. The diet of early humans was much lower in fat, very rich in vitamin C and contained many times the amount minerals such as magnesium, calcium and potassium of the modern human diet.

Early humans also ate much more fiber, which is virtually absent in meat. "Although the practice of adding some amount of meat to the regular daily intake became a pivotal force in the emergence of modern humans, this behavior does not mean that people today are biologically suited to the virtually fiber-free diet many of us now consume," according to Katharine Milton,[17] professor of physical anthropology at the University of California in Berkeley. "In fact, in its general form, our digestive tract does not seem to be greatly modified from that of the common ancestor of apes and humans, which was undoubtedly a strongly herbivorous animal."

Our closest living relatives, extant apes (including chimpanzees, orangutans and gorillas)[18] are skilled at capturing live prey, particularly monkeys.

However, they prefer insects as their main animal protein source. They derive about 94% of their calories from plants, leaving about 6% from animal sources. They also consume abundant wild fruit that is more fibrous than cultivated fruit that we buy in supermarkets. So they end up consuming hundreds of grams of fiber every day, while the average American eats about ten grams per day.

Dietary fiber positively affects sex hormones[19] and lowers insulin levels.[20] Excess fat and estrogen is passed out of the body through the digestive tract, with the help of fiber in our diets. Eating more fruits, vegetables and other fibrous foods assists this process.

Those who do not have enough fiber in their diets have much higher rates of estrogen-related breast cancer. In one study, for example, they measured the weight of female poop, to see how much fiber they were getting, and compared that with rates of estrogen excretion. The heavier poo indicated higher fiber in the diet, and those with higher fiber had more efficient elimination of excess estrogen via the bowels.[21]

In patients with polycystic ovarian syndrome,[22] combined dietary fiber and magnesium improved insulin resistance and improved androgen levels. Soluble fiber increased satiety hormones when ingested with a meal.[23] Eating abundant fresh fruits and vegetables is a great strategy for getting lots of fiber in the diet.

Vitamin D

Low T? More like *Low D*. Vitamin D is great for your D. or V. It's great for all body parts related to pleasure, and then some. That's because a.) it's not really a vitamin but a hormone our body makes from sunlight, and b.) without it, sex simply won't be as good.

The hot sun on our bodies nourishes the body with qi, or vital energy, warming the kidney yang, which is the seat of sexual fire. Vitamin D plays an integral role in calcium homeostasis within the body. Yet vitamin D deficiency is a huge problem, affecting about 1 billion[24] people worldwide and leading to a host of issues that put a damper on getting down.

First, deficiency is associated with increased blood pressure and cardiovascular disease risk. The heart has to work harder, and those with deficiency suffer higher incidence of sudden arrhythmic death.[25] It stiffens arteries (ironically, not penises) and causes vascular dysfunction. Hypertension also lowers available nitric oxide, which is associated with less pleasure and sexual response for everyone.

Males with the lowest levels of vitamin D had a two-and-a-half times greater risk of heart attack. In fact, a large portion of patients with cardiovascular disease have low levels of vitamin D. Adequate vitamin D levels are also associated with lower blood pressure and lower incidence of stroke.

Increased vitamin D from sunlight decreases arterial calcification, a risk factor for erectile dysfunction (ED), and raises levels of free testosterone. Remember that free testosterone in the body is that which is unbound and available for use, what we want for hot sex.

Higher vitamin D levels reduce excess blood sugar and improve insulin resistance. It also counteracts inflammation, which is a major player in reduced sexual pleasure and ED.[26]

Because low vitamin D is associated with poor sexual function, some people began taking vitamin D supplements. Some of these people found however, that this resulted in even worse sexual function. That's because taking vitamin D can worsen a pre-existing magnesium deficiency.[27]

I recommend getting vitamins from whole food sources, and vitamin D from sunlight. Of course, anyone with a diagnosed deficiency may want to supplement and should work with their physician. As little as twenty minutes outside at mid-day a few times a week can provide plenty of vitamin D, though this isn't always possible in the winter. But again, we can eat our way out of this problem in numerous ways, for example, oyster mushroom and other mushrooms are a great source of dietary vitamin D[28] in winter months, and I'll include more recipes at the end of the book.

Cruciferous Vegetables

Brassica, also known as cruciferous vegetables, include things like broccoli, cabbage, arugula, red radish, cauliflower, Brussels sprouts and collard greens. Ironically, your date might need a gas mask at first, but they're great for your junk. In research, these vegetables demonstrated a significant benefit to the endocrine system and should be a staple of the diet in preventing non-communicable diseases such as obesity, Type 2 diabetes, cancer and a variety of other chronic illnesses, all of which affect pleasure in the bedroom. Brassica vegetables have detoxifying properties, anti-carcinogenic effects and anti-inflammatory properties.

Cruciferous vegetables are rich in phytonutrients and minerals which promote health and protect nerves going to and from the genitals. As such, they are central to the great sex diet. These vegetables are high in polyphenols, vitamin C, sulfuric compounds, such as sulforaphane, as well as glucosinolates (GSLs) and 3,3'-Diindolylmethane (DIM), which improve health by preventing obesity, protecting nerves and reducing inflammation in your body.

In patients with ovarian cancer, DIM-treated subjects had 1.5 times better chance of staying cancer-free because it inhibited the cancer precursor cells. Still other research demonstrated that DIM reduced breast tumor markers.

Cruciferous vegetable consumption can reduce some markers of inflammation in healthy adults,[29] and is associated with a decreased risk of prostate cancer.[30] Sulforaphane, a sulfuric compound in cruciferous vegetables, has demonstrated anti-oxidant, anti-inflammatory, anti-cancer properties. In addition to killing prostate cancer cells,[31] it reduced PSA levels in some males[32] and positively altered gene expression.

Sulforaphane also improved cardiac function by inhibiting oxidative stress and reducing inflammation.[33] Because of these anti-oxidant properties, it showed in research ability to protect the male reproductive system in obese subjects, improving sperm count and motility, and decreasing insulin resistance.

Phenethyl isothiocyanate (PEITC) is another substance found in cruciferous vegetables. In research it reduced hyperplasia of prostate cells[34] and improved hormonal balance.[35]

It's easy to incorporate more brassica in the diet. Cooking methods affected the content of various nutrients[36] with some nutrients being more bioavailable when eaten raw and others activated by steaming. For this reason, you can go both ways. Simply add them to salads, steam them or make them your centerpiece. After tackling the dietary strategy I gave her, Carla's favorite is a Tuscan kale potato soup (recipe included), which is truly delicious.

B Vitamins

B vitamins—found abundantly in fresh fruits and vegetables—are essential for great sex. They are involved in cellular energy and metabolism and exert a great influence on both sex hormones and nerves. Increasing dietary B vitamins have been shown in research to affect levels of testosterone and improve sexual function. B vitamins are essential for proper nerve conduction to and from the genitals. They protect nerves against the effects[37] of oxidative stress, which slows signals for less pleasure in adults.

Good sources of B vitamins include:

- Nuts and seeds
- Salmon
- Mushrooms
- Legumes
- Peanuts
- Mangos
- Avocados
- Green peas
- Yams
- Potatoes
- Green vegetables
- Spinach
- Asparagus

Do **not** take megadoses of B vitamins, as this has been shown in research to cause nerve problems, which is the last thing we want for pleasure.

There is quite a bit of research demonstrating the role of B vitamins in male sexual health. Unfortunately there is a severe lack of research on B vitamins and female sexual health. This doesn't mean that it's not just as important. It just means that scientists and researchers don't pay as much attention to female sexual function since they tend to assume that a functioning vagina trumps whether sex was good for us or not.

Thiamine, Vitamin B1	This B vitamin plays an important role in nerve conduction, as well as muscle and heart contraction. It is also involved in carbohydrate metabolism. Thiamine and B6 deficiency causes peripheral neuropathy. Studies found that sluggish nerves due to thiamine deficiency were corrected by simply administering thiamine.[38] Thiamine plays a significant role in reproductive health. As males age, they tend to produce less sperm and sex hormones. In the testicles, aging is associated with atrophy (degeneration) of tissues. In research, thiamine decreased testicular atrophy in aging males and improved sexual function. Further, it increased testosterone levels, antioxidant status and increased overall sexual activity.[39]
Riboflavin (Vitamin B2)	Riboflavin is highly concentrated in sperm. It has been found to be protective against oxidative stress,[40] which benefits blood vessels and nerves. Additionally, it reduces the risk of certain cancers. In female bodies of menstruating age, it is necessary for reproduction and deficiency can disrupt sex hormones, leading to infertility.[41]
Niacin (Vitamin B3)	Vitamin B3 was shown in research to improve serum testosterone levels and antioxidant status in male diabetic testes.[42] Niacin reduces circulating FFA (free fatty acids) and increases GH (Growth Hormone). In patients with moderate to severe erectile dysfunction, and dyslipidemia, niacin alone improved erectile function.[43] Iron, niacin, folate and B12 have also been shown to boost dopamine, which also affects sexual pleasure.
Pantothenic acid (Vitamin B5)	Pantothenic acid (vitamin B5) is a panty dropper and has been shown in research to be an essential factor in sex hormones, testicular function and sperm quality.[44] In female bodies, it has been shown to be important for reproductive health.
Vitamin B6	For fast nerves, and optimal testosterone, get adequate B6, which significantly improved nerve conduction velocity in diabetic patients.[45] Deficiency causes significant testosterone disruption in males.[46]

Folate (Vitamin B9)	Better folate than never (or too soon)! Research has shown a significant correlation between folic acid deficiency and erectile dysfunction.[47] Other studies have indicated that low folic acid is a risk factor in premature ejaculation and erectile dysfunction.
	There is a strong relationship between serum folic acid levels and sexual function. Males with ED, PE or both had lower folic acid levels than healthy subjects.[48] One study, for example, found that, in patients with diabetic neuropathy, taking a folic acid supplement significantly improved the speed at which nerves sent signals.[49]
Vitamin B12	The vitamin B12-Bomber is essential for the production of myelin, the insulating sheath that covers nerves and ensures that they fire quickly and strongly to and from the genitals. For this reason, those who are deficient show diminished nerve function[50] in research. Optimal nerve signaling to and from the genitals is a crucial aspect of sexual function and pleasure.
	B12 intake was associated with a slight increase in testosterone in females, as well as a reduction in homocysteine, which is a risk factor for heart disease.[51] Vegans and vegetarians have higher homocysteine levels (though lower rates of heart disease), due to lower levels of vitamin B12.[52] Vegans and meat eaters alike are at risk of low vitamin B12. In fact, about 39% of meat eaters are in the low-normal range for blood concentrations of this vitamin. Studies have shown that both deficient and low levels cause worse sensory and peripheral nerve function[53] and impeded growth of dendrites[54] (nerve "arms").
	B12 is involved in spermatogenesis, or the production of sperm. Research demonstrates that vitamin B12 increases sperm count, enhances sperm motility and reduces damage to sperm DNA.[55]
	For vegans, B12 must be taken in the form of a supplement, but for meat eaters, you'll find it in fish and meat. However, since subclinical B12 deficiency is so widespread,[56] some would benefit from supplementation.

Fasting

Fasting makes the nasty so much nastier. Don't be put off by the concept of fasting as you've likely heard about it, typically a starvation crash diet that feels like, well, starving. When done intermittently and responsibly, it confers numerous health benefits and creates a lightness, restfulness and overall wellness that sets the stage for better sex.

Traditional Chinese medicine takes a much gentler approach, believing in eating during the yang cycle, or daylight, and fasting during the yin cycle, or night. This gives the digestive organs much-needed rest.

Fasting has deep historical roots and is, after all, part of every major world religion. Jewish people fast on Yom Kippur and six other minor fast days of the year. Mormons fast for two consecutive meals on the first Sunday of each month. During the month of Ramadan, Muslims fast from sunrise to sunset. Hindus on the new moon, and Buddhists on the full moon. Ancient people recognized not only the spiritual benefits but the health benefits of fasting.

Periodic or intermittent fasting has been found to improve cardio-vascular disease, diabetes, cancers, neurological disorders and stroke. It also helped people to lose weight and improve insulin sensitivity. Fasting improves metabolic function in non-diabetic patients as well.

On a cellular level, fasting improves mitochondrial health and DNA repair.[57] It promotes autophagy, which is a process by which cells clean out the garage, getting rid of distorted and impaired cellular molecules and structures.

Fasting has consistently shown in research to lengthen life expectancy and reduce the risk of major diseases. It does so by signaling pathways that slow aging and disease processes,[58] enhance performance and optimize physiological function.

Fasting and Oxidative Stress

Fasting also reduces the production of pro-inflammatory substances by our bodies and boosts antioxidant activity. It diminishes oxidative stress to endothelial cells, boosting bio-availability of nitric oxide, which is great for blood flow to the genitals and also for pleasure.

For these same reasons, fasting is protective against atherosclerosis, decreasing cardiovascular risk and mortality.[59] Fasting reduces fat tissue mass, reduces blood pressure, heart rate and improves our lipid profile. It decreases cholesterol, increasing HDL and lowering LDL. When we care for the vascular system, we assist the delivery of blood to the genitals. Remember, this is just as important for female sexual function as it is for males.

Fasting decreases waist circumference, which is associated with improved insulin sensitivity. It also reduces stress and depression and improves self esteem.[60]

Fasting protects nerves from degeneration.[61] This makes nerves fire stronger, faster impulses to and from the genitals for better function and more pleasure.

Fasting, Hormonal Balance and Sexual Function

Overnutrition results in disruptions in LH, FSH, leptin and insulin levels. Fasting increases adiponectin, which promotes insulin sensitivity and weight loss. Humans with long lives have higher levels of this protein.

Research demonstrates that fasting improves reproductive and mental health. It reduces stress hormones[62] and increases LH in obese females with PCOS to correct ovulation issues.

DHEA (dehydroepiandrosterone) is a precursor of androgens such as testosterone in males and females and plays an important role in sexual function and responsiveness. DHEA normally declines with age, but calorie restriction offsets this decline.[63]

Intermittent fasting raises testosterone levels in male and female subjects.[64] A study published in JAMA tracked people reducing calories by 25% for two years, finding that sexual drive and relationships improved significantly compared with those not restricting calories.[65] Other studies found that fasting increased weight of male testes[66] and enhanced growth hormone release.[67]

Studies have shown that even a single period of fasting reduces metabolic biomarkers associated with chronic disease such as insulin and glucose.[68] Additionally, fasting positively affects thyroid hormones.[69]

So, How Do I Fast?

First, anyone should consult a physician before starting a fasting schedule, but, in general, I recommend once a week for twenty-four hours. That means no food but plenty of water or herbal tea. This is much easier to do if you make your fasting window from dinner to dinner, because you're only skipping breakfast and lunch one day.

Let's say your fasting day is Wednesday. That means that after dinner on Tuesday, you would not eat anything for the rest of the night. Then on Wednesday, you would not eat until dinner, though you would still drink water and herbal tea throughout the day. This method is particularly suited to those who have a difficult time going to bed hungry.

It's typical in the first week of trying this to discover that you eat more at dinner than normal, but as your body acclimates, you will find that you eat only slightly more than a normal dinner in future weeks.

To be clear, I **do not** recommend more drastic forms of fasting as outcomes are not favorable. Prolonged fasting in Chinese medicine is believed to weaken our digestive spleen qi, which in many ways corresponds to the human microbiome. For females, research shows that severe caloric restriction shuts down reproduction. In males,[70] long term, severe calorie restriction reduces total and free testosterone.

Putting It All Together

All this is to say that Carla and Dan found that taking the time to prepare meals at home and eat more whole foods was the best strategy for a great sex diet. Instead of getting breakfast on the go, Dan made himself a green smoothie with spinach and berries most days. For lunch, Carla made sure to include lots of vegetables, such as a baked yam with steamed broccoli and a salad. As a result, they were getting much higher quantities of necessary nutrients for great sex such as B vitamins, antioxidants and minerals.

Every Wednesday, each of them would fast for twenty-four hours with no food from 6 p.m. Tuesday until 6 p.m. Wednesday. After a few weeks of adjustment, they found that it was relatively easy to forgo breakfast and lunch, which also spared them the time of meal prep. Their hormones shifted for the better as a result, and vegetables replaced refined sugars in their diet.

And then, boom: Their bodies were able to launch a strong physical response to sexual arousal, which meant harder erections for Dan and abundant blood flow and lubrication for Carla. When your body works that well, your brain has less time for stage fright. Chapter 14 contains lots of delicious recipes to incorporate these dietary recommendations.

Summary of Diet for Hormonal and Sexual Health

Yin and yang are the way of sex. To maintain their delicate balance for optimal pleasure and function, we must eat well. A lower-fat diet, while getting adequate vitamin D, fiber, B vitamins and leafy greens, promotes hormonal balance. In addition, brassica vegetables contain various phyto-nutrients which promote sexual health. Research also supports the use of brief periods of fasting to help normalize hormones.

When we nourish both the cool feminine yin and the hot scorching male yang within ourselves, the essences of sex are at their finest. Yin and yang in harmony brings the ecstasy and excitement of heaven and earth reunited in passionate sex.

THE NERVOUS SYSTEM AND GREAT SEX

Nora had a long list of comically embarrassing dating stories that sounded like something straight out of a *Cathy* comic. The latest: She had been stood up on Valentine's Day for a romantic dinner by a guy she'd already slept with, and now she found herself standing directly in front of him in line at the grocery store.

She'd imagined running into Henry before, but in her preferred scenario, she would be dressed to kill, a devoted beefcake on her arm, preferably in a sleek convertible. Reality, however, was less the revenge fantasy she'd hoped for and more of a sad trombone. She was disheveled, alone, bloated from recent weight gain, and just as she noticed him noticing her, the yeast infection treatment on the conveyer belt she'd grabbed rolled in mortifying slow motion toward the cashier.

Nora wasn't exactly *surprised* that he wasn't interested. The sex was bad. Their first night together he came in under two minutes, then had the gall to complain that *she* took forever to get off. And even though she knew such jabs were mere declarations of insecurity, she still felt like it was somehow her fault. Nora vowed in that very moment that she would have better sex with a better guy.

When I met Nora, she had just started dating someone new and was hoping to get her body in shape sexually. She didn't want to give the Henrys of the world an easier time, but she wanted her body to feel as responsive as possible.

I treated Nora with acupuncture and dietary intervention to move her closer to that holy trinity: healthy nerves, improved vascular function and hormonal balance. The goal was to make her clitoral nerves more sensitive to stimulation, so she would have an easier time orgasming. In the beginning she noticed subtle improvements, and after a few months sex was a whole different experience.

Of course, Henry had a different way of seeing things, as Nora later discovered. He was just as mortified in line at the grocery store. The first time they were together, it had been a while since he had had sex and Nora had gotten him extremely horny. As a result, he came in two minutes. He knew this was pretty common for the first time with someone, but then Nora laughed and called him the minute man.

To avoid this, he tried masturbating before their next date so he could last longer. But that led to a second, equally wince-inducing sad trombone moment: Nora, excited to get it on immediately, was all over him the second he was in the door, and having just jerked off, but unable to say so out of embarrassment, he presented a flag flying at half-mast. He ditched on the relationship rather than face his embarrassment at having disappointed Nora.

I treat many male patients in my acupuncture practice who simply want to last longer, so I place needles in various places throughout their bodies, including the fleshy area below the tailbone. This is where the sea of yang begins. The yang is what ignites lust and the qi that holds ejaculate until the right moment. By stimulating the nerves in this area, patients report stronger erections and better ejaculation. In addition to diet, this reinforces the trifecta of sexual health—nerve, cardiovascular and hormonal health.

Acupuncture promotes health by moving qi, or vital life force, along the meridians of the body. Blocked or insufficient qi causes disease, so we move the qi to improve sexual function. The qi is the key.

This traditional Chinese view has been verified by modern science. The meridians correspond to the vascular and nervous systems. The nervous system exerts control over every chemical substance produced by the body. This includes all hormones and neurotransmitters such as testosterone, estrogen, nitric oxide and dopamine. The nervous system consists of the brain, spinal cord and nerves. The penis, testicles, vagina and clitoris are abundant with nerves.

While most of us don't know how strongly our nerves fire, much less realize their essential role in orgasm, this process is a critical aspect of great sex. Research clearly shows that stronger, faster nerve impulses make for better sex. Again here, the Chinese were ahead of their time, for they understood this concept thousands of years ago. A strong qi flowing through the vessels is needed for sexual function. From arousal to climax, the qi influences pleasure.

The food we eat drives how quickly and strongly our nerves fire. For the best sex, we should incorporate certain foods into our diet which protect and nourish the qi. High antioxidant foods are a great choice, and mushrooms, for instance, with their very high antioxidant content, are able to improve the human microbiome to an impressive degree.

But foods that are fatty, rich and heavy, particularly processed foods, slow the qi. So every time we eat dinner at the vending machine, we are slowing our sexual qi, which makes for less-pleasurable sex.

Qi, Nerves and Sex

I treat patients from both a biomedical and traditional perspective. Biomedically, we work toward optimizing that holy grail of great sex: vascular, hormonal and nerve function. Traditional Chinese medicine strives simply for balance of yin and yang. Developed before microbiology or radiography, it uses natural phenomena to explain the complex biological processes of nerve and vascular function. This is where balancing hormones and eating for optimal sexual health comes in: We feed yin and yang through our diets, behaviors and even emotions.

What's really happening when we get horny? As simple as it seems, arousal, sex and orgasm are a complex system of input and output acting in sync. Imagine that your partner touches you, their hand tracing from your stomach down between your legs.

As their palm and fingers touch your skin, they stimulate nerves with distinct pathways on your abdomen and genitals. This electric impulse takes that story to your spine and hopes it answers the door when it comes a knockin'. It reflexively triggers arousal, with blood flowing to the genitals. The impulse also calls to the brain, where lust is ignited.

In a complex chemical sequence, areas of your brain release dopamine, which is pure chemical pleasure. The brain also responds with nerve impulses to our genitals, strengthening our arousal response: vaginal lubrication and an influx of yin blood to the vagina, clitoris or penis.

When clitoral and penile nerve stimulation reaches its threshold, a flood of dopamine ensues, resulting in orgasm. Similarly, your eyes and nose have nerves that communicate with the brain when you see an erotic site, like your partner's naked body, or even simply smell their fragrance.

Structures in your brain *understand* this stimuli as sexually arousing and respond accordingly. Even our thoughts and memories alone can activate parts of the brain that will cause sexual arousal. But success always hinges on how effectively those response mechanisms are working.

You can also view this from a traditional lens. The emotions of being with your partner activate the heart, liver and kidneys. Their touch ignites the lusty yang qi, which squeezes blood vessels, propelling the yin blood through the arteries to the mysterious gate, the clitoris, vagina or penis. Yang builds continuously until climax, and then transforms to yin. Sexual pleasure, then, relies on the yang qi, or proper nerve conduction.

Some nerves go from the genitals, to the spine and travel up to the brain. Other nerves go from the genitals to the spine and never go to the brain to be processed. Instead, in a reflexive action, pathways from the spine return straight to the genitals.

That's encouraging news for those whose qi is physically blocked because it demonstrates how adaptable our bodies can be in spite of roadblocks in the midst of this complex process. Studies of male soldiers who suffered spinal cord injury in World War II, for example, found that most were still able to achieve some erection, and some were even able to climax. Similarly, about 50% of females with a spinal cord injury were still able to orgasm.[71]

Nerve Health and Sex

Given the connections between hormones, sensation, blood flow and great sex, it's easy to see the importance of the vascular system, which houses the blood that fills our genitals. But without proper nerve conduction, our genitals will not fill with blood, making orgasm impossible. A large percentage of females[72] and males[73] with sexual dysfunction have weaker nerve signals and slow nerve conduction speed.

One study found that in 105 males with erectile difficulties, nearly all were associated with vascular issues or nerve conduction problems. In fact, *half* in total had sluggish nerves![74] The sexual experience for females operates in the same way. When nerves fire slowly, they feel less pleasure and have trouble achieving orgasm.[75]

When we care for our nerves, they reward us with sensation. What this means sexually is that:

- Situations that should be arousing will result in strong nerve impulses signaling sexual arousal.
- When the genitals are stimulated, our nerves will send strong signals to and from the spine.
- Signals arriving to the brain will be correctly processed as intense sexual pleasure.

The stronger this signaling process, the more pleasure you feel. By caring for our nerves, we ensure proper nerve conduction. Many factors can affect this process, but a high-fat diet, chronic illnesses, and aging, for example, will all slow nerves and reduce sexual pleasure.

Back to Nora. Her high-fat, low-carbohydrate diet had led to neuro-degeneration. This is a progressive loss of nerve structure and function, which may eventually result in nerves dying off entirely. Nora's nerves were sending weak, unreliable signals between her genitals, spine and brain, which is why orgasm was so difficult for her. In traditional Chinese terms, her rich, cloying diet was slowing and blocking her qi.

Scientists have discovered that problems with nerve signaling result in a reduction of available nitric oxide to the smooth muscle in the genitals. Simply put, that means less sexual pleasure. Erections are less firm, and the clitoris becomes less responsive, leading to reduced arousal. It also leads to the formation of collagen within the smooth muscle tissue of the genitals which further blocks the qi. I use herbs in my practice to move qi, which have shown in research to increase the production of nitric oxide.[76] Again, ancient Chinese physicians knew what they were doing without even a course in microbiology.

Some of us find that the older we get, the more difficult it can be to get off. As we age, one study found,[77] our nerves impulses are weaker and slower, and take longer to respond to stimuli. What this means for sex is that communication between the genitals, spinal cord and brain is not as good, resulting in less arousal and less pleasure. Older people who ate more antioxidants and omega 3s, though, had much better nerve conduction.[78] Other foods also improve signals to and from our genitals.

This means that we can still encourage optimal response even as we get older. We can help our nerves to fire beautifully by nurturing them with the very food we eat. And for those of us who already have great sex, here is a way to ensure that we will continue to for a very long time to come, which dovetails nicely with the greater skill and comfort we experience in sex as we get older.

How Does Food Affect Nerve Conduction and Sex?

Food can be the best sex therapy we'll ever find. It nourishes the qi and keeps it flowing freely. It dictates how well our nerves send signals to and from the genitals and to our brains. Certain foods make nerves send signals more quickly, with a stronger magnitude. They generally do this by protecting nerves from oxidative stress, as well as helping to rebuild and repair damage.

Food also affects nerve signaling by influencing levels of neurotransmitters, which are the chemical communicators between nerves. According to Dr. Richard Wurtman, professor of neuroscience at MIT, the nutrients in food are the building blocks of chemicals produced by our bodies.

Not surprisingly, they are affected by how much or how little of those building blocks we eat. Selenium, folic acid and other B vitamins, which we will discuss in other chapters, have all been shown to affect levels of neurotransmitters such as serotonin and dopamine. Antioxidants protect nerves from damage and improve speed and strength of nerve signals. It follows that we should be eating foods high in key nutrients and importantly, antioxidants.

Antioxidants

Diet affects sex. At this point, you may wonder why, as teenagers or younger adults, you recall such a guaranteed lusty sexual experience no matter what you ate. I'm with you there. As a teenager, I recall one instance where the "romantic dinner" I prepared for my boyfriend one night when my mother was away consisted of a frozen chicken dinner and some Rice-A-Roni containing zero fruits or vegetables. I didn't have much game in bedroom or in the kitchen, and had no idea what an antioxidant was, but it certainly had no impact on our eagerness and enthusiasm to experience each other.

The fact is, a sixteen-year-old's body can usually take this kind of abuse in the short term. But as we mature, all that dietary fat has a cumulative effect on nerve and arterial function. Had I known then what I know now, I could've have prepared something off my menu for great sex, which you can see in Chapter 14. But it definitely would have included lots of antioxidants, which are truly one of the most important nutrients we can take into our bodies. Here's why:

An antioxidant has an anti- in front of it because it prevents what's in the second half of the word: oxidation. So it follows that an antioxidant is a substance that prevents genetic changes and injury to DNA in cells caused by oxidation. Oxidation is a complex chemical process resulting in damage to our tissues, such as blood vessels and nerves.

But all you need to understand is that oxidation makes nerves fire sluggishly. Antioxidants, on the other hand, encourage nerves to fire quickly and strongly. They help to keep the qi unblocked and free-flowing. *This* is what we want as our partner touches us. *This* is how we in turn feel pleasure. We want nerves that can accurately tell the story of what's happening in our heads to the rest of our bodies. This strong signaling causes the maximum reaction in our bodies and minds, and all we have to do to help them is feed them well.

We know from research that by increasing antioxidants in the diet, we significantly reduce oxidative stress to nerves. That increases nerve conduction velocity,[79] for better sex, and benefits even those of us carrying extra weight. Though excess body weight can slow nerves, so could the diet of a rail-thin person living off burritos and sodas. Weight is not the whole picture. Antioxidants can still help in either scenario. Vitamin E, for instance, is a powerful antioxidant that has been shown in research to speed up sciatic nerve velocity in obese subjects.[80] I'm not here to lecture anyone on a specific weight, but rather to show how maximum healthfulness in diet will ensure these connections remain intact, and ideal weight, which is always individual, tends to find a better balance as a result.

Research has also shown that antioxidant supplementation protects the testes and sperm against the harmful effects of environmental toxins such as cadmium, lead, industrial pollutants and radiation.[81]

Much of the damage to blood vessels in the penis and clitoris is the result of oxidative stress. Eating fatty, salty meals causes oxidation and reduces the release of nitric oxide within penile and clitoral arteries. However, consuming antioxidants has been shown in numerous studies to blunt damage to blood vessels.[82]

Again, traditional Chinese medicine was ahead of its time in understanding that antioxidants are a kind of insurance policy against poor sexual function. Herbs used in Chinese medicine such as Hawthorn fruit and Salvia have been shown in research to effectively treat sexual issues.[83] Not coincidentally, they both have a very high antioxidant content.[84]

Examples of antioxidants include vitamins:

- A
- C
- E
- Beta-carotene
- Lycopene
- Lutein
- Selenium
- Manganese

And compounds known as polyphenols, such as flavonoids and Alpha-Lipoic acid. Where can we find antioxidants in the foods we eat?

Polyphenols: Polyphenols are a type of antioxidant found in many fruits and vegetables. There are several types of polyphenols, which have been shown to improve cardiovascular health. Two important types are flavonoids and phenolic acid.

Flavonoids: Flavonoids are found in many fruits and vegetables. Numerous studies have demonstrated that flavonoids in certain foods are good for heart health and erectile function. Additionally, flavonoids are good for vascular endothelial function. This is the innermost layer of the walls of blood vessels.

Flavonoid-rich foods include:

- Onions
- Apples
- Berries
- Kale
- Leeks
- Broccoli
- Blueberries
- Parsley
- Fresh citrus fruits
- Celery

What is even better than flavonoids or nitrate-rich foods for sex? Both of them combined! One study compared healthy people eating apples (flavonoid-rich), spinach (nitrate-rich), or both apples and spinach, to control subjects. Both apples and spinach benefited arterial function, but spinach combined with apples lowered blood pressure more than either by itself. And you don't have to eat these foods for years to see a benefit. Measurable improvements are observed in blood vessels shortly after eating them.[85]

Phenolic Acid: Berries, apples and cherries are good sources of phenolic acid, which has been shown clinically to improve elasticity of blood vessels, which typically decline with age. This elasticity is critical to delivering blood to the penis, vagina and clitoris, and ultimately leads to sexual pleasure.

For Nora, I recommended she eat berries with nuts every morning for breakfast instead of her usual eggs, bacon and toast, or yogurt. Not only was she caring for her nerves, making them more sensitive to her partner's touch, but she felt more energetic throughout the day. As a result, she noticed she was no longer too tired for sex at night as she had been in the past.

Food Sources of Some Common Antioxidants

Vitamin A	Vitamin C	Vitamin E	Polyphenols	ALA
Orange fruits and vegetables such as carrots, butternut squash, cantaloupe, apricots and peaches	Countless fruits, vegetables and mushrooms are great sources of vitamin C such as berries, citrus, potatoes, papaya, peppers, tomatoes and broccoli	Nuts, seeds, mango, avocado, leafy greens, squash, mushrooms, fish and red peppers are great sources	Tea, citrus fruit, berries, apples, walnuts and legumes are all great sources.	Walnuts, chia seeds and flax seeds are all good sources.

MUSHROOMS, NERVES AND GREAT SEX

Antioxidants help nerves send more pleasure signals to and from the genitals, and many foods are rich sources. But what if I told you mushrooms, which are loaded with antioxidants, will do much of the heavy lifting? Both a food and a medicine, they are the motherlode of foods, and confer near-magical status for the health benefits they offer. That's why they are at the top of my list.

I know, I know, mushrooms aren't for everyone. Some of my patients despise mushrooms — the rubbery texture, the earthy taste. They aren't swayed by their amazing health benefits. I tell them they just haven't tried enough of them yet, nor do they understand the myriad ways they can be consumed, even for the texture- and taste-averse. You can eat them, you can drink them, you can bake them, you can pickle them. To my knowledge you can't snort them — to be clear, I'm not talking about psychedelic 'shrooms here — but when it comes to mushrooms, anything is likely possible, and my fingers are crossed we can some day absorb them through osmosis, IV or at least topically (again, the food kind).

I do have a secret mushroom weapon for the timid: I fell in love with chaga mushrooms, and recommend trying the chaga chai latte (recipe included). This tends to seal the deal for my mushroom haters, primarily because chaga, with its natural vanilla flavor, is delicious, and no pesky texture problem.

There are about 140,000 species of mushrooms in existence. Ancient Chinese physicians regarded these beautiful organisms as an elixir of immortality and a symbol of luck and well-being. There are loads of mushrooms prescribed in traditional Chinese medicine. Poria, for example, is a solid white fungus that grows around the roots of pine trees and is used in innumerable traditional herbal formulas. Reishi and wood-ear mushrooms taste great in a soup. Research has documented antimicrobial, antiviral, antiallergic, immunomodulating, anti-inflammatory, antiatherogenic, hypoglycemic and hepatoprotective properties of various mushrooms.[86] It can't be overstated that finding a way to work mushrooms into your diet will be great for your sex life. *Got mushrooms?* should be the rallying cry of the sex health industry.

Microbiome

Perhaps understanding how mushrooms pull this magical status off will help persuade you. To grasp how they are capable of achieving so much in the body, we must understand the role of the human microbiome in health and in sex. What is a microbiome? Our unique microbiome is comprised of communities of microscopic organisms, existing everywhere in our bodies, from our stomach and intestines to our eyes, ears and skin.

These organisms, including bacteria, fungus, viruses and protozoa, can either live in harmony with our bodies or act as pathogens. They can improve our health or diminish it, affecting our risk of a great number of diseases, obesity and even anxiety.

To illustrate, let's take a look at one such study[87]:

Group A were subjects at high risk of cardiovascular disease. Group B were healthy subjects with average risk. Researchers transplanted the feces of group A to the intestines of group B. Following the transplant, group B too developed high risk of cardiovascular disease.

What happened? The microbiome of group A was transferred to group B, indicating that even cardiovascular disease risk depends on the types of microbes that live in our bodies. Some microbes increase risk while others protect us. You get the point, even if we're talking feces here.

Interest in the human microbiome has exploded (no fecal study pun intended) in the last decade, and for good reason. Clinical trials have produced undeniable evidence that most aspects of human health depend on the balance of microbes living in our bodies. Without very specific microbes, our bodies cannot produce or absorb many nutrients. And when microbial populations are unbalanced, disease takes the opportunity to spread.

A balanced microbiome is one component of a strong spleen qi. In Chinese medicine the spleen qi is what transforms our food and drink into the essences of the body. Our immune system and the qi of the entire body depend on healthy spleen qi, which commands all body fluids, including genital blood flow.

How do we get our microbiome?

Well, you can't buy it on Amazon. The first microbes to colonize our digestive tract come from our mothers at birth via our passage through the birth canal (in case you wanted one more reason to blame her, but don't, she gave you the good stuff). Our heads and mouths pass through her vagina, ingesting vaginal secretions, bacteria and small amounts of feces. Interestingly, research has shown that babies born via C-section have microbiomes reflecting hospital microbes, while babies born vaginally have microbiomes like their mothers.[88] This affects the caesarian babies' immune systems, for these children suffer from increased childhood allergies, asthma and autoimmune disease.[89] Later on, our diets[90] affect our microbiome, as do the use of pharmaceuticals, pathogens,[91] antibiotics,[92] exercise[93] and lifestyle.[94]

We also pick up microbes from the fruits and vegetables we eat, which also have distinct bacteria that tends to grow on them. Organic and conventional produce differ in the bacteria found growing on their surfaces, and we are exposed to these microbes when we eat these raw. Different diets and even exercise also affect microbial populations in our gut.

In addition to weight management, diabetes, heart disease, inflammation and hormonal health, the human microbiome also affects nerve health,[95] blood pressure, stress, anxiety and sex hormones. Great sex, from a physiological standpoint, is the coordinated effort of strong, rapid nerve impulses and healthy blood vessels, all influenced by balanced sex hormones. All three of these components are affected for better or worse by the balance in our microbiome. In fact, some prominent microbiologists have advocated for the development of products that treat sexual dysfunction by shifting microbial populations in the gut.[96]

Here's where Amazon could come in: Because of its considerable effect on human health, all sorts of products have been developed to increase beneficial microbes, such as probiotics. Most probiotics at this point in time, however, do not colonize the intestines and offer limited benefit. But mushrooms — even simple white mushrooms that you find in the grocery store or could order online via grocery delivery — actually do alter the human microbiome. This in turn, improves our sex lives.

Mushrooms, the Microbiome and Sex

To put it mildly, mushrooms positively effect on our microbiome. Their true benefit is more like a slam dunk: They promote healthy nerves, blood vessels and hormonal balance, i.e., that holy trinity of great sex I won't shut up about. Their very high antioxidant content I mentioned also makes mushrooms anti-aging, providing a more youthful appearance, hotter body and better cognitive function, all things that will make anyone feel better, even in the dark, and even in a bar at last call.

Mushrooms act as a prebiotic, meaning they feed the healthy microbes in the intestinal tract. Researchers have found that mushrooms contain prebiotic substances such as polysaccharides like chitin, hemicellulose, β and α-glucans, mannans, xylans, and galactans. All sorts of mushrooms, from white mushrooms to exotic shiitake, turkey tail and lion's mane, positively alter bacterial flora in the digestive tract in clinical trials.[97]

While they're all superstars, each mushroom actually has a unique effect on the body, demonstrating an ability to treat obesity, increase insulin sensitivity, reduce blood lipids (fats) and maintain nerve health.[98]

All that said, some of these mushrooms are exotic to standard Western grocery stores. But you don't have to get unfamiliar mushrooms outside of your typical shopping list. Even eating simple, white button mushrooms found in any supermarket will significantly benefit your health. They have the same inflammation-reducing,[99] immune-system boosting, anti-bacterial properties as the others, and they still increase microbial diversity in the gut.[100]

And they aren't just a boon for gut health, but also the nervous system. Nerve inflammation leads to degeneration of nerves, but mushrooms reduce nerve inflammation and even *reverse* oxidative damage in the brain.[101] In research, culinary mushrooms promoted nerve growth[102] and prevented nerve death.[103] Mushrooms have also been used to effectively treat infertility due to testicular damage.[104]

But that's not all! Mushrooms, as I promised, play every part in that trifecta of great sexual health, so they also strengthen our cardiovascular system. They lower blood pressure, cholesterol and reduce the risk of stroke in numerous studies.[105] And as you know now, cardiovascular health is a major player in sexual health.

I got Nora into mushrooms, and as she was dedicated in her pursuit of great sex, she found recipes to her liking so that she now eats them almost daily. Her preferences: sliced in salads, and cooked with potatoes and onions for a mushroom hash. Science would say that these mushrooms are transforming Nora's gut health, but all she knows is that she is having better sex. Bonus: There are no more Henrys to hide from at the grocery store.

A Few of My Favorites

Every human being is an exquisitely crafted work of art, each with our own species of genius to bestow upon the world. So too are mushrooms. If there's a place to experiment on occasion and incorporate less familiar but more powerhouse mushrooms into your diet where possible, let a few of my favorites be your guide. These could be found in Asian markets, health food grocery stores and upscale grocery stores with a wider selection.

Reishi Mushrooms

In addition to their powerful benefit to the immune system, Reishi mushrooms have demonstrated their ability to repair damaged nerves, rebalance sex hormones and improve mood, all important factors in sexual health. Several studies have found that they fight obesity by positively affecting gut microbes associated with healthy weight.[106]

In one study, obese subjects were given a water extract of Reishi mushrooms for eight weeks. They lost a significant amount of weight during this time, and markers of inflammation were markedly reduced. They then transferred the feces of these subjects to the intestines of a new group of obese subjects. They were able achieve the same results, even though the new group of obese subjects had not taken Reishi mushrooms.

What this means is that Reishi mushrooms helped the subjects lose weight by changing their gut flora.[107] This is important to sexual pleasure because being at an unhealthy weight often disrupts sex hormones. Obesity-related inflammation also slows nerves, resulting in less pleasure for everyone.

Shiitake Mushrooms

Shiitake mushrooms are particularly flavorful and loaded with benefits to sex. Used in Asia for thousands of years medicinally, they have been shown to protect and repair nerves in several studies. Shiitake mushrooms also have essential amino acids, B vitamins and loads of trace minerals like selenium and zinc, which strengthen and repair nerves. They also have the ability to ward off pathogenic viruses and bacteria.

Turkey Tail

Turkey tail mushrooms have proven in research to possess anti-tumor, anti-inflammatory, antioxidant[108] and antibacterial properties. They are also used in many integrative cancer treatment centers to inhibit the growth of cancer cells and stimulate the immune system. Turkey tail mushrooms both protect nerves and help repair damage to them.[109] Turkey tail also improves the way cells use oxygen, leading to better stamina in the bedroom, exercise performance and reduction of fatigue.[110] In one study, a turkey-tail-based vaginal gel improved microbial quality in the vagina and improved vaginal health.[111]

Lion's Mane

Many nerves are covered with a fatty substance called myelin. Similar to the insulation on electric wires, myelin is extremely important for nerve protection and conduction. When myelin is damaged, nerve signals can't move as quickly and so nerves don't fire properly. Lion's mane, among other mushrooms, encourages myelin creation.[112] It also protects against stress-induced nerve cell death.[113] Reishi, hen-of-the-woods, bitter tooth fungus and lion's mane mushrooms have all been found to benefit nerves and the brain in this way.

In research, lion's mane and tiger milk, for example, both protected nerves from injury. And even more impressive, these mushrooms encouraged regeneration of damaged nerves.[114] Healthy nerves send the strongest, fastest nerve impulses to and from the genitals for the best sex. I like to add lion's mane, oyster mushrooms and plain white mushrooms to my Sunday sauce (recipe included) and serve it over spaghetti.

Cordyceps

Don't sweat that cordyceps is a fungus that grows parasitically on caterpillars, killing its host. Embrace it because it enhances the way our cells use oxygen. Used to boost performance and energy, it is also anti-viral. Cordyceps, which promotes longevity, has been used in China for over 2,000 years for great sex.

Several recent studies have demonstrated measurable improvements in libido and desire in subjects. Cordyceps increased testosterone in males and significantly improved sperm count and sperm quality.[115] In one study,[116] reishi and cordyceps significantly improved endurance in athletes, raising testosterone and reducing the stress hormone cortisol while cycling after three months of supplementation. Other mushrooms too, have demonstrated ability to positively affect sex hormones in the body.[117]

Cordyceps also protects against oxidative stress,[118] benefits cholesterol and lowers triglycerides. It is also a natural vasodilator, which increases blood flow to sex organs.

Chaga Mushrooms

Remember my secret mushroom weapon? There are lots of tasty ways to incorporate mushrooms into our lives, but for those particularly hesitant, I recommend chaga. Chaga grows on birch and other trees, embedding itself in the bark and emerging as a large black knot.

Because of its pleasing vanilla flavor, chaga was used as a coffee substitute during World War II. Woody chunks of the mushroom are boiled until the water becomes caramel-colored, just like coffee. It can be served plain or with honey. If you want to elevate it, you can make a chaga chai latte (recipe included), iced or hot, with almond milk, cardamom, cinnamon, nutmeg and fennel. The chaga chunks can be dried and reused several times. I like to make a big pot of it and have it over the course of a few days. Wild harvested chaga can be purchased on Etsy or Amazon.

Abundant in antioxidants, chaga is antiviral, anti-tumor and anti-inflammatory. In one study, chaga lowered blood sugar in diabetic patients in just three weeks. In another study,[119] its antioxidant effects boosted the immune system by significantly reducing damage to DNA in lymphocytes. Chaga benefits the heart by improving cholesterol levels and reducing levels of triglycerides (fatty substances associated with stroke) in the blood. These accumulations are a physical manifestation of qi blockage.

**

If your grocery store doesn't carry these mushroom varieties, try specialty stores. As noted above, Asian markets, health food stores, farmer's markets or upscale grocers carry a wider variety of fresh mushrooms, and if there's an Asian market in your area, the cost difference may be negligible or in your favor. In Wegman's, a more upscale chain in the Northeast and mid-Atlantic, for example, I often find fresh lion's mane and oyster mushrooms, which are a wonderful addition to soups and sauces.

Alternately, you can sauté mushrooms and serve them over salmon, potatoes or really *anything* savory. All they need is a sprinkle of salt and are a wonderful addition to meals. You can also use mushrooms as the base for many dishes instead of meat. For example, I shredded some mushrooms and used it as the basis for a Chipotle-style sofritas (recipe included). I made a delicious burrito bowl out of this and topped it with fresh guacamole and salsa.

You may be tempted to use some of those mushrooms growing in your backyard, but make sure you know your mushrooms before doing something like this, as many are poisonous.

What NOT to eat for optimal nerve function

While front-loading our bodies with the good stuff is essential to a great sex diet, so is avoiding foods that derail the very healthy efforts we're making for improvement.

Growing up in the '80s, pretty much everything I ate came from a box. I was raised by a single mom who was always working two or three jobs, so dinner was Dinty Moore beef stew in a can or TV dinners like Salisbury steak and fried chicken. And there was the dubiously named Suddenly Salad!, which wasn't salad at all but pasta drenched in oil and salty seasonings.

Those were the days. You could really enjoy shitty food without thinking about all the damage it was doing to your body. I had no idea that all that fat and salt were damaging the nerves in my clitoris, or that it could affect my ability to orgasm later on. Not until I was much older and concerned about my own pleasure in the bedroom did I even consider the effect of food on my sex life.

For great sex, qi and blood must be able to flow freely through the vessels. Rich, cloying foods block the vessels and result in less pleasurable sex. Generally speaking, heavily salted, fatty and processed foods should be avoided in favor of fresher, lighter foods.

Too much fat in the diet slows the qi. Many studies have confirmed what the Chinese have known for millennia: Eating a high-fat diet can slow nerve conduction and make nerve signals weaker. This directly equates to less-pleasurable genital stimulation and sex that isn't as good. So, when touched or rubbed, the penile or clitoral nerves sending information to the spine and brain are slower, which is not what we want for maximum enjoyment.

As we talked about earlier, dopamine is a neurohormone very much involved in human sexual arousal, motivation, performance and orgasm. Numerous studies have found that eating a diet high in saturated fats disrupts dopamine signaling in the brain. Simply changing our diet can improve or even reverse damage caused by high fat. Caring for our nerves, just as caring for our blood vessels, requires keeping fat intake low.

I've seen numerous patients transform their sex lives by making better food choices. A thirty-nine-year-old patient named William, for example, had his prostate removed. This procedure often severs nerves associated with sexual function, causing impotence. His surgeon was able to spare his nerves in the procedure, but even so he sometimes lost his erection during sex, which led to frustration and embarrassment.

William drastically reduced his fat intake, substituting more fruits and vegetables, including a salad every day for lunch. He balanced rich, heavy yin foods with light, airy yang foods. He also incorporated lots of lion's mane mushrooms, and he liked to top his salmon with them. After several months, William rarely lost his erection, and as a result, had better sex.

Summary

Sexuality is a delightful part of the human experience for many of us. At our best we are kind, purposeful and altruistic, and when our bodies are cared for, we are also horny. No matter our age or health, our identity or orientation, we are biologically wired to connect physically with others and are built with channels connecting our genitals with our minds.

For the hottest, most responsive, satisfying sex, we must nourish the qi and keep clear its path by limiting fat. As commander of the blood, the qi likes powerful protectors loaded with antioxidants like mushrooms, berries, mangos, walnuts and countless other fruits and vegetables. A healthy qi arises from a robust microbiome, a living army dutifully supporting its commander, a storyteller whose path is cleared to send the loudest, strongest message. In a body that is well nourished, where qi and blood move freely, desire comes to us naturally, pleasure comes to us naturally, and orgasm is effortless.

THE VASCULAR SYSTEM AND GREAT SEX

After weeks of dating, tonight was the night Tasha and Debi would finally take things up a notch. Tasha was ready with a sexy setup: She'd prepared two steaks, opened a bottle of her finest red, and lit a few candles for mood. From her vantage point, nothing could go wrong.

As they made out on the couch, Debi took the lead, moving her hands slowly down Tasha's body as she removed her clothes. Tasha was eager and excited to finally get physical with Debi. It had been a while since Debi was with a partner, so she was extremely into this. She always left her lovers flush in the afterglow of pleasure, and hoped Tasha would be the same. She and Tasha had a real connection, and she could see a future with her.

Tasha lay there, knees apart, when Debi suddenly reached to put her glasses on. She put one hand on Tasha's knee, and with the other hand, reached inside as if she was fishing something out of the drain, squinting.

Tasha froze. *Is she looking for lost jewelry? Why does she need her glasses? Has this girl ever seen a vagina before?!* It seemed like lately, though, no one she dated seemed to know what the hell they were doing down there.

Debi, unfazed, felt sure that her partner would soon be making the O face. But when she glanced up at Tasha, she looked more like she was praying for a pap smear to wrap up. *Why wasn't her signature move working!?*

Embarrassed and inhibited, neither of them climaxed that night. Tasha and Debi continued their relationship, but it was a struggle in the beginning to get each other off. Tasha thought that Debi was unskilled, and Debi thought that Tasha was unpleasurable.

Only that wasn't the whole story. In reality, none of Tasha's lovers could please her in recent years because she had poor blood flow to her genitals, interrupting the very pathway to responsiveness that great sex depends on.

She had Type 2 diabetes and high blood pressure, which can damage blood vessels. And if you've been paying attention, damaged blood vessels simply can't deliver adequate blood to the vagina and clitoris. And if the blood isn't flowing, the O isn't coming.

What's more, everyone seems to remember that erections depend on that crucial blood flow, but we forget that it's equally essential for female arousal and pleasure. For Tasha, this thwarted pathway explained precisely why she had difficulty not just getting off, but also connecting to Debi's touch sensually during foreplay.

I treated Tasha with acupuncture to course-correct and get her blood flowing to her genitals. Acupuncture, need I remind you, stimulates points on the meridians of the body, through which qi and blood flows. These meridians correspond to the vascular and nervous systems of the body.

I inserted needles in various parts of her body, including the perineum, which is the fleshy area located between the anus and the vagina or scrotum, and a key erogenous zone, too, as it's a major crossing point of nerves associated with sex. In TCM terms, this is where the sea of yin begins. The cool, feminine yin essence is the blood and fluids that fill the vagina, clitoris and penis.

Debi would learn some new tricks, too, and together they would address diet as a main prescriptive toward better sexual health. As they both grew more comfortable with each other's bodies, and drastically changed their eating habits to boost their vascular and sexual health, things started moving. They now have great sex and laugh about the comedy of errors in their early dating.

TCM for TCB

Ancient Chinese medicine, radically ahead of its time, understood all this. Qi and blood must flow freely for proper sexual function. Blockage of the vessels causes stagnation of bodily substance, letting disease run amok, messing with the very connections that responsiveness depends on.

So in treating reproductive function, acupuncture, Chinese medicinal herbs, and Chinese dietary therapy all serve a single goal: to nourish the free flow and abundance of the essences of sex because good blood flow is critical to great sex for everyone.

To assist this, we give our bodies the raw materials to maintain the integrity of blood vessel walls and to repair damage. Second, we keep them clear of accumulation—the tiny blood vessels of the penis and clitoris are easily blocked with plaque, which can make for less pleasurable sex and weaker erections.

The food we eat does most of the heavy lifting. Caring for our penile and clitoral arteries involves keeping fats low and eating the right types of fats. These blood vessels also require appropriately balanced minerals, including a low salt and adequate potassium diet.

Foods, such as spinach and beets, with their naturally high nitrate content, protect blood vessels and promote vasodilation for increased blood flow to the genitals. Eating abundant antioxidants, which is discussed in the previous chapter, also greatly protects the vessels of sex.

There Will Be Blood

When we talk about incredible sex and powerful orgasm, we have to talk about blood. Or rather, the vascular system, what it's doing, and how to feed it. This may not sound like pillow talk, but being horny is essentially blood flowing freely and abundantly to your junk. We don't have to think about a horny bloodbath when we're in the moment (unless it's that time of the month), but when we experience magnificent sexual pleasure and toe-curling orgasms, that's your blood talking. (More like shouting, with glee.)

We make the blood go where it needs by eating foods that send it on its merry way instead of slowing it down to a sluggish, non-horny stop. Our bodies are brilliant machines that can chomp on a snack, extract its essence, or essential qi, and from this generate blood. Then, the blood picks up the torch and runs it directly to all the tissues of the body, and when the mood hits, makes a pit stop in our genitals for a little fun. It cannot be overstated that we *must* care for these vessels through proper diet.

What we eat is essential to this process of sending nutrient-rich blood to the right places, even in those of us who are in great physical shape. That's because we can see vascular damage already in healthy people showing no signs of cardiovascular issues.[120] That's right: Nearly all of us already have visible plaque accumulating in our arteries by the time we finish high school. Researchers discovered this when doing autopsies on young adults who had died in accidents or in war and found that nearly all of the young people they examined had early coronary heart disease, only it was still too mild at that stage to cause heart attack[121].

The point here is that when we become aroused, that's blood doing its thing. Blood engorges the penis for males. Blood engorges the vagina and clitoris for females. This increase in blood volume in turns leads to vaginal lubrication, creating the feeling of wetness that signals arousal. How does it do this? Because when we are turned on, the nervous system releases nitric oxide (NO) and acetylcholine, stimulating the increase of a substance called cGMP and causing arteries in the genitals to fill with blood. (Try dropping that little tidbit next time you're at a singles bar.)

Take Viagra, typically thought of as an insta-horny boner pill that takes a man from standby to liftoff in minutes (and tragically, sometimes for hours). Only, Viagra does not actually *cause* sexual arousal, rather it improves blood flow to the penis (keeping those cGMP levels high), which in turn makes the blood vessels more responsive to sexual excitement.

But if it were really just a pill for boners, then why does it have the same affect on women? Because of blood. Some studies testing Viagra on female bodies found that it significantly increased vaginal lubrication and blood flow to the clitoris.[122] It also increased arousal, and 57% reported that the clitoris had improved sensitivity.[123]

Blood flow is blood flow, no matter the parts, and when blood flows, arousal skyrockets.

Eat, Pray, Bone

Again, here's where nature lends a helping hand. Lots of natural foods increase nitric oxide levels, causing vasodilation and more elasticity, some-times even just within a couple hours. Researchers have documented changes in how well blood vessels work even after a *single* meal.[124]

This means there are quite literally *sex foods*, not just as a celebratory meal before diving into bed to give our blood vessels a boost, but as fuel for the entire trip. When we eat these foods, our arteries will deliver more blood to our sex organs for a night of lovemaking. The magnitude of effect in the short run may be less than the boost from a pill, but changing dietary habits will lead to better, sustained sex over the long haul so that our metaphorical and literal boners can crank themselves. And you won't have to worry about showing up at your doctor's office with your four-hour boner.

Let's Talk About Fat, Baby

You may not believe me, but McDonald's is a great place for dietary guidance. I used to go there with a friend who liked their $1 coffee, and sometimes we'd have to pull over and wait for a fresh pot. There was a tree on the side of the parking lot, and under it, a brown plastic garbage bin where customers could toss their trash.

While waiting one day for her cup of joe, I spied a squirrel rifling through the garbage. At a glance it looked like any cute squirrel I'd seen gathering nuts in the park, but then…I actually got a look at it. This squirrel was rocking love handles and a fat ass. It would waddle down the tree, into the garbage, then, a moment later, emerge with food, hauling it back up for a nosh. It struggled through this process several times, and on repeat visits, I checked back in on its adventures, equal parts amused and horrified.

Then it struck me. This squirrel kind of looked like me, like a lot of people hanging around McDonald's, and like many Americans.

Typically, animals in the wild naturally eat what's right for them, and their tastes reflect nutritional requirements. Outside of domesticated pets we overfeed, you just don't see animals watching their figures, trying to cut calories to get that bikini body. They don't need to. They eat the right food for their physiology, which naturally promotes healthy body shape, optimal health, and hot sex.

But just like us, when fresh and nutritious isn't around, they eat what's available and convenient. And for this squirrel, that was McDonald's. This squirrel's eerily human physique was proof that when animals eat like typical Americans—that is, fatty, salty, processed food—their bodies protest, too.

This is instructive. Eating fatty food stiffens our blood vessels, which makes our heart work harder. Even after one fatty meal, such as chicken and cheese, according to one study, the blood vessels become measurably stiffer within a mere few hours.[125] We want our blood vessels, arteries and veins to be more elastic because blood is then able to move more freely, giving our heart a break. Free-flowing blood, as you recall, means free-flowing orgasm.

Think of it this way: If you were feeling a little randy, would you watch something erotic to rally the forces or queue up a tearjerker and dampen the mood? You'd rally the forces, of course. Similarly, foods can enhance the mood for love or kill it (or at least slow it down to a comically sad degree), and it's up to us to direct our troops to battle with a victory mindset.

High fat stagnates qi and blood in the du, ren and chong mai, which are the meridians of sex I told you about. It causes accumulation in the vessels and thickening that hampers the ability of vital sex essences to travel to our genitals. In scientific terms, we call this hyperlipidemia, when there is too much fat in the blood, caused directly by a high-fat diet. Female patients with hyperlipidemia have significantly lower arousal, lubrication, orgasm, and satisfaction.[126] A very high-fat diet is associated with imbalance in weight, and unfavorable hormone changes.[127]

But nature is healing. Even after damaging blood vessels with high fat, simple changes in diet can help normalize blood flow to the genitals[128] again with the right protocol.

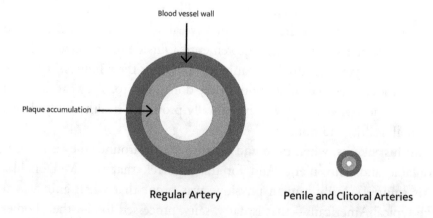

Blood vessel wall

Plaque accumulation

Regular Artery   **Penile and Clitoral Arteries**

Penile and clitoral arteries become obstructed before other arteries because of their size.

Fatty foods don't just stiffen blood vessels, they also cause plaque build-up. Because the blood vessels going to the penis[129] and clitoris[130] are some of the smallest in the body, they'll be the first to take the hit. For instance, long before a person sees signs of heart disease, they will notice that sexual pleasure and function[131] decline.[132] Males who are diagnosed with ED in their forties are also about fifty times more likely to develop coronary artery disease.[133]

Plaque accumulation, in turn, restricts that precious blood flow, making it all the more difficult for the clitoris to become fully engorged with blood. This is called clitoral vascular resistance, wherein your clitoris basically becomes a conscientious objector, protesting against the food you've fed it by refusing to feel anything. The more weight we gain, and the more insulin resistant we become, the more clitoral resistance increases.[134] Simply put, it means less blood flow and we know what that means now: less female pleasure. Less responsive to touch. And if you can't feel it, you can't come.

Speaking of clitorises in revolt, back to Tasha. Tasha, as noted, suffered from Type 2 diabetes, which damaged her blood vessels. I inventoried her eating habits and discovered she ate meals out most days, and takeout tends to be higher in fat (and sodium). That didn't help the arteries and nerves leading to and from her clitoris, which became more sluggish. This in turn meant her arousal response was poor. In other words, her rich, cloying diet was blocking the flow of qi and blood, and all this was blocking her ability to fully feel and respond to Debi's touch.

To get her clitoris out of the dumps, Tasha had to quit feeding it like it was a garbage can. She had to change her diet, which can actually reverse damage to blood vessels caused by excessive fat intake.[135] Reducing daily fat intake may not sound hot, but at least it's a simple formula. The recommended daily allowance (RDA) of fat is sixty grams, but if you are in good health, striving for forty is an excellent and worthy goal.

Reducing plaque in the arteries requires a *bit* more reduction of fat. Here, researchers found that it was possible to reduce arterial plaque accumulation with a diet comprised of about 10% of calories coming from fat, and abundant fruits and vegetables, especially leafy greens.[136] In a 2,000 calorie-per-day diet, this would be twenty-two grams of fat per day.

I've treated many patients, male and female, who seek treatment when blood vessels are partially occluded and beginning to show signs of revolt in the form of sexual decline.

One patient, Travis, had noticed recently that his erections weren't always as firm as they had been, and he had been diagnosed with high cholesterol and high blood pressure. He was in his late thirties and wished to aggressively improve sexual function and show his penis who's boss.

As such, he reduced his fat intake by two thirds and incorporated more fruits and vegetables, especially spinach, into his diet. He began to notice sexual improvements almost immediately, and after five months, his erections were consistently so strong they were practically saluting him.

The Fat-Sugar Combo

If too much fat does a number on our blood vessels, then eating high fat *plus* high sugar is a particularly lethal combination. Even just consuming *one* high fat-high sugar meal results in immediate low-grade inflammation in our bodies and havoc in our blood vessels.[137] Though this is a temporary state, when we chronically challenge our bodies with high fat and high sugar we continually assault our blood vessels, making it more difficult for them to do their job.

Mind Your Ps and Os

Before you take all the fats in your cupboard out back and shoot them, a plot twist: Not all fats do the walk of shame. Fats regulate the production of hormones in the body, so healthy hormone balance requires some of this stuff. But it's the amount of fat, and the type of fat, that makes all the difference.

Each type of fat has a unique chemical structure which effects our bodies differently. Polyunsaturated fatty acids (PUFAs) and omega 3 fatty acids are among the healthiest for sex. They are found in nuts, seeds and fish.

Reducing saturated fat lowers the risk of heart disease, but you can't just replace saturated fat with carbohydrates, especially refined ones. That won't reduce vascular damage. We need to replace saturated fats with polyunsaturated fats to reduce the risk. And while we're at it, replacing some carbohydrates with PUFAs found in fish, seeds and nuts will also reduce the risk of CVD.[138]

In males, fat intake, especially PUFAs, was significantly correlated with total and free testosterone levels. In healthy females,[139] increased PUFA intake was associated with very small increases in testosterone.

Omega 3 fatty acids, also found in oily fish, nuts and seeds, offer tremendous benefit to us in the bedroom through their action on both the vascular system and on our nerves. Many studies have demonstrated signs of improved cardiovascular health and endothelial function by eating a diet rich in omega 3 fatty acids. For this reason, I recommend including them in my patient's diets.

Omega 3s are yin in nature but without being as cloying and qi-slowing as other fats, which is why they are so popular in modern health literature. There are different types of omega 3 fatty acids including EPA (Eicosapentaenoic acid) and DHA (Docosahexaenoic acid), found primarily in oily fish, and ALA (alpha-linolenic acid), found in nuts and seeds such as walnuts, chia seeds and flax seeds. The human body can convert ALA to EPA and DHA. (Quick, say that backwards.)

All you really need to know is that these acids are very important for your blood vessels and for the other sex organ we've neglected to mention until now: your brain.

This Is Your Brain on Fat

If you think our genitals are having all the fun when we get it on, imagine what's going on upstairs. Your brain is the master organ of your sexual function, involved in all successive steps of your sexuality, and it is having a field day. It is also about 60% fat. Twenty percent of that fat is made up of essential fatty acids. Your body cannot make omega 3s though. They must be obtained from what we eat.

DHA, highly concentrated in the cerebral cortex, testes and sperm, makes up a huge portion of the fats in the brain, where our body doles out pleasure. As such, omega 3s are key in how the brain functions, playing a part in neurotransmission, inflammation, oxidation and even how genes express themselves in the brain.[140]

DHA, present in brain cell membranes, is necessary for nerve cells to talk to each other, with dopamine being the key messenger. Higher dopamine levels are associated with greater arousal and sexual behavior.[141] Studies have shown that a diet low in omega 3 fatty acids results in decreased dopamine in the frontal cortex of the brain, where a great deal of sexual processing occurs.

A Little Mood Music

Given this association with dopamine levels, omega 3s, especially EPA, are quite handy in reducing anxiety and depression.[142] Sex hormones can affect levels of DHA in areas of the brain associated with mood. Females suffer from major depression at a rate twice that of males, and the reason for this, aside from the stressors of being a woman these days, is that it may be linked with deficiency in omega 3 fatty acids secondary to a dysregulation in ovarian hormones.[143]

Translation: Eat more Omega 3s already, would you?

Please Get on My Nerves

Omega 3 fatty acids don't stop there. They also reduce oxidative stress on nerves, essentially serving as an antioxidant.[144] In research, they upgraded how nerves fire in the brain[145] and sped up nerve conduction in the rest of the body.[146] This effect was seen both in patients with damaged nerves and in healthy subjects.[147] Omega 3s also affect electrical currents and other cellular functions of nerve cells.[148] Sexually, this translates to better sexual response when our genitals are stimulated or our minds are aroused. They make you hornier, okay?

Acetylcholine, another neurotransmitter found in the brain that's fun to discuss at parties, is involved in arousal and male and female sexual responses. Eating more omega 3 fatty acids calibrated acetylcholine in the brain[149] and got those nerves talking better than ever.

Baby-Making Boost

Want to breed? Omega 3s are your new best friend. Dietary omega 3 fatty acids affect female reproductive health, improving the quality of eggs and extending their reproductive lifespan.[150] Omega 3 from marine sources was associated with higher progesterone levels and reduced risk of anovulation (failure to ovulate, a cool T-shirt slogan, but not so cool for would-be parents). Females who increased dietary intake of PUFAs improved metabolic and endocrine characteristics.[151]

For males, studies have found that, even following serious penile nerve injury, subjects given DHA had significantly stronger erections.[152] Omega 3 fat intake was associated with higher testicular volume, while higher omega 6 fatty acid intake was associated with lower testicular volume.

Trans fats (you'll find them in cookies, donuts and other processed foods) are associated with lower testosterone levels. Higher omega 6 (found in processed foods) intake is associated with higher LH levels, the luteinizing hormone that, when lower and balanced, aids in reproduction in ovaries and testes.[153]

Repeat After Me: Fish, Nuts, Seeds

We can make sure we're getting enough PUFAs and omega 3s by eating fish, nuts and seeds. Chia seeds count. Flax seeds count too. Both contain quite abundant quantities, so you only need a very small amount. Some forms of algae are rich in omega 3s, so if you're looking for a supplement, choose an algae-based one. Getting enough in your diet is easy though, as delicious choices such as salmon, walnuts and avocado abound. Moderation is key here, so while oils also contain these beneficial fats, they are very dense and high in calories. Oils should be limited in favor of nuts, seeds and fish.

Fish

Fish, fish, fish. They get all the attention, are always picked first for dodgeball, and are perennially flacked as the greatest source of omega 3s. Apologies, but I love fish and I'm here to flack fish once more: Healthy people who eat fish at least twice a week have less plaque build-up and less vascular inflammation. Which means they have better sex. Fish eaters also age better, as the fatty acids in fish were found in studies to prevent damage to DNA. Eat more fish.

I have some bad fish news, too, though! Fish can contain higher levels of harmful metals such as arsenic and mercury. That said, other, better fish are still the answer to the bad fish. Wild salmon (yep, it's a fish) is a good choice in that it has high levels of omega 3 fatty acids, which is what is good for your blood vessels (and genitals!), and lower mercury levels. You don't have to eat a ton of fish! Just sticking with a three to four ounce serving a couple times a week is a good choice.

My patient, Tasha, drastically reduced her intake of fat by cutting out baked goods, cheese and processed foods. Instead, she cooked at home more and began to include—you guessed it—fish in her diet a couple times a week. She noticed surprisingly quickly that her clitoris was much, much happier with her and less prone to outbursts. She had more clitoral sensitivity when Debi touched her. As a result, arousal and orgasm came much more naturally, and Debi was happier with her too.

Minerals

Reproductive function is highly dependent on minerals, nature's little spark plugs.

They are involved in a vast number of bodily processes. Calcium, magnesium, iron, copper, zinc and selenium are all helpers for cardiovascular, endocrine and nerve health, and that means they'll help you get laid better.

In the female reproductive cycle, minerals influence hormones which control processes such as ovulation. Copper, for instance, can induce ovulation[154] following stimulation of the hypothalamus. Not getting enough iron is associated with ovulatory infertility.[155] Some minerals can even induce ovulation by serving as an antioxidant, effectively controlling oxidative stress, which has been proven in research[156] to reduce fertility.

In males, minerals' fingerprints are all over your testicular health and sperm quality, and the male body needs a proper mineral balance to calibrate the production of androgens such as testosterone.

In the West, we struggle to eat appropriate quantities of protein, carbs, fat, vitamins and minerals. Traditional Chinese medicine, though, guides us to optimal mineral nutrition by eating a balance of yin and yang and the five flavors: sweet, sour, acrid, bitter and salty.

Sodium

We need it. We're obsessed with it. Too much is bad. Too little is bad. Whereas low sodium intake shifts hormonal balance in the wrong direction, with lower concentrations of progesterone, so does too much sodium. When one flavor among the five is overrepresented, as salt is, it disrupts the delicate balance of yin and yang. For optimal sexual function, we should be eating less than a teaspoon of salt per day.

Too Much Salt, Too Little Potassium*[1]

Too much salt and too little potassium makes Jack a very dull boy. Jill, too. We're all screwed when we have too much salt, and not in the way we'd like to be. Some 99.4% of Americans consume too much salt. Even more alarming, over 90% of us consume more sodium than is even considered tolerable for human consumption![157] You don't have to know that for your body to do a double-take when you overdose on it. Even a single salty meal can impair arterial function within thirty minutes, reducing nitric oxide release,[158] which is critical for arousal.

Of note, some theories suggest that our kidneys flush out all of the excess salt in our diets, so we shouldn't sweat the intake. This isn't entirely true. Yes, our bodies maintain very precise levels of sodium and potassium in spite of what we eat, but this comes at a price, one that demonstrates how much potassium and sodium are linked.

When you eat a salt bomb for a meal, first, your kidneys have to excrete potassium to get rid of the excess sodium. That might be no big deal if we had enough potassium on hand to aid in this delicate internal carwash, but we don't. Historically, we used to consume about ten times as much potassium as sodium in our diets, but now it is just the opposite: We take in about ten times more sodium than potassium.[159]

So, while we're eating too much sodium, which is causing high blood pressure and damaging blood vessels (ah yes, those things again), our kidneys are knocking themselves out trying to conserve the potassium we do have. It does that through reabsorption, and that is a tiresome process, requiring a lot of energy.[160] We could definitely use that energy somewhere else. Ideas, anyone?

Poor potassium intake is not just bad for blood vessels in the short-term, either, it's the gift that keeps on giving. Potassium softens the vascular endothelium (the very important inner lining of blood vessels) and increases nitric oxide release shortly after consumption.[161] And, as we've already talked about, we want that nitric oxide for something else, for

---

* Certain groups of people, such as those with kidney disease, may have to limit potassium intake, and should consult their doctor on appropriate intake.

more blood flow to the genitals and better sex. We don't need to outsource it to the kidney carwash.

According to recent medical literature, 98% of Americans do not get enough potassium (though I'd love to meet that 2%). This leads to vascular calcifications, which are mineral deposits on the walls of our blood vessels, which can stick to fatty plaque that is already present there. As you rightly suspect, this is not good for bringing that crucial blood flow to the clitoris and penis.

So. Easy answers: Increase potassium intake. That will counteract the calcification of blood vessels, making them become more pliable and reducing blood pressure.[162] This will get to work fixing those blood vessels[163] and reduce the risk of cardiovascular disease. And also, it frees your body's resources up for things it actually enjoys doing—nothing against carwashes.

Potassium Sources

Quick, name a source of potassium that isn't a banana. I'll wait. If you didn't say yams and squash, orange you glad I didn't say fish? Er, moving on: Great sources of potassium include:

- Potato
- Yam
- Squash
- Cantaloupe
- Fig
- Kiwi
- Mango
- Orange
- Pomegranate
- Artichoke
- Avocado
- Leafy greens
- Broccoli
- Pumpkin
- Banana

First thoughts? You may have noticed from this list that it's difficult to get enough potassium if you're not eating a lot of plants. Bingo. One study measured the effect on blood vessels of increasing potassium by adding one baked potato and two bananas to the diet every day. Guess what function improved? Blood vessels.[164]

Don't point the finger at potatoes. They have been unjustly vilified in the low-carb and keto movement, which suggests to me they're not doing great personal PR about the fact that they also assist in great sex. Yes, potatoes. Good for doing it. Who knew?

Okay, there's a catch: We're not talking about French fries or greasy, loaded baked potatoes. We are talking about simply prepared potatoes as part of a low-fat diet. Potatoes, and their misunderstood cousins, yams, are some of the best sources of potassium, not to mention other important nutrients.

Potassium is so important for good sex that I advise a potassium-rich meal for two-hours before having it. Studies show an immediate, measurable improvement in vascular endothelial function after just one high-potassium meal.[165] Hey, it's good enough for athletes, who depend on it to balance fluids and aid in muscle contractions for the big competition. And sex, after all, is an endurance sport.

Tasha and Debi got hot for potassium. Well, more accurately, they started having a banana and berries with walnuts for a delicious breakfast every morning. Then, for dinner they often ate pan-seared salmon and yam or baked potato. In addition to better sex, they lost weight along the way, and now have more energy than before.

Calcium for Shagging

There are only four other elements more abundant in the human body than calcium, which for our purposes makes it the Fifth Element of sex. It is essential for muscle contraction, communication between cells and nerve transmission. Our bodies don't make it though, so it must be obtained from the diet.

Calcium plays a starring role in hormonal secretion, as low vitamin D and calcium are associated with reduced sperm motility and total sperm count as well as lower testosterone.[166] In females, our bodies naturally shift calcium, magnesium and phosphorous levels during different times in our menstrual cycles.[167] Low calcium intake is associated with reduced proges-terone levels.[168]

Higher calcium buffers against cadmium exposure,[169] which I mention because heavy metal exposure impairs sexual and reproductive function.

Calcium, along with isoflavones, vitamin D and inulin improved sexual function, body composition and metabolic parameters in menopausal women. Specifically, desire, subjective arousal, lubrication, orgasm and satisfaction all increased.[170]

Worth noting: Some experts have advised *against* taking calcium supple-ments regularly because they found in research that they slightly, but significantly, increase the risk of heart attack[171] and strokes. That needn't trouble us, as there are plenty of safe and delicious ways to get calcium from our diets, including leafy green vegetables, broccoli and nuts, such as almonds.

Magnesium, P.I.

Another mineral, another tale of deficiency. Americans only get about 50% of adequate dietary magnesium, which is a bummer because it just so happens to be involved in over 300 metabolic processes in the body. A few cases where magnesium is the mineral for the job? Muscle contrac-tion, nerve conduction and cardiac function,[172] as well as blood sugar and insulin, which are all important for sexual pleasure and function.

Low magnesium is associated with a host of bodily woes, such as stress, fibromyalgia, chronic fatigue syndrome and headaches. Deficiency leads to nervousness, and even psychosis, and can cause anxiety and depres-sion. It elevates risk of stroke. Low levels are associated with hypertension, cardiovascular disease, stroke, migraines and attention deficit hyperac-tivity disorder (ADHD).[173] We need it for optimal nerve transmission and neuromuscular coordination.

But when you calibrate it correctly, it delivers. Adequate intake reduces risk of Type 2 diabetes as well as cardiovascular disease.[174] It boosts anti-oxidant activity to reduce oxidative stress and increases mitochondrial effi-ciency. It is also essential for muscular and cardiac contraction and release.

We also need it to make DNA and RNA, as well as regulate metabo-lism and insulin metabolism. Those who eat a high magnesium diet have better insulin sensitivity,[175] while low magnesium intake is associated with Type 2 diabetes and metabolic syndrome.[176] Getting enough means lower fasting insulin levels and less insulin resistance, indicating better sugar metabolism.[177]

Magnesium[178] also has a hand in stress, buffering cortisol production, and too little lowers testosterone, which can diminish both male and female sexual function.[179] In research, magnesium supplementation had beneficial effects on male gonads.[180] Similarly, progesterone is known as a female hormone, but it is also critical in the production of testosterone.

It is difficult to say what the optimal amount of magnesium intake should be, and there is a great deal of debate about this. The RDA is 350 milligrams, but if you look to other primates such as monkeys, their intake is closer to 1300mg[181] due to their larger intake of leaves and fruits, suggesting we might be able to safely go a bit above the RDA in our diets.

Plants, again, are your friend: They're a great source of magnesium in nuts, pumpkin seeds, legumes, white potatoes, fish, sunflower seeds, cashews, figs and spinach.

Think Zinc

Zinc is found in all human cells and is a major player in male and female sexual health, and yet again we don't get enough of it. In order to survive, our bodies work to maintain a constant state of cellular zinc. Zinc deficiency is a worldwide problem, affecting even the well-fed US population. Some studies estimate that about 50% of Americans are not taking in adequate quantities of zinc.[182] However, one recent study,[183] reported much higher, estimating that 98% of Americans have a zinc-deficient diet.

Regardless, our bodies desperately need it. Zinc promotes cardiovascular health and reduces arteriosclerosis,[184] lowering our risk of cardiovascular disease.[185] Zinc appears to have antioxidant effects[186] and deficiency leads to cellular damage and atherosclerosis.[187] Zinc is anti-inflammatory[188] and reduces risk of numerous infections, including pneumonia.

As for sexual function, it's a humdinger. Much research has linked zinc to fertility in both men and women. Without enough zinc, sperm production,[189] testosterone production and ovarian and testicular function all suffer.

But research suggests zinc supplementation or simply adequate animal protein can correct some of this. For males, as little as three months of supplementing saw a 75% increase in testosterone. In females, Zinc supplementation improved sexual function at certain doses. When given too much though, it impaired sexual function.[190]

How we get zinc in our diets is important: Grains and legumes are a great source, with a caveat. There are substances in grains and legumes called phytates, which inhibit zinc absorption by the body. Because of this, soaking, sprouting or fermenting the grains and legumes—historically a common practice until more recent times—will reduce or virtually eliminate phytates, making zinc more bioavailable.

Several studies have shown that protein will boost zinc absorption because the amino acids in protein keep zinc in solution, which increases it bioavailability.

Manganese, If You Please

Female bodies need manganese in particular to keep the cycle running smoothly: levels below 1.8mg/day were associated with increased risk of anovulation, failure to ovulate in a given menstrual cycle.[191] Manganese and iron levels were significantly lower in females with polycystic ovarian syndrome (PCOS).[192] Sources of Mn are nuts, legumes, yams, spinach and whole grains.

Selenium Falcon

Certain enzymes involved in menstruation need selenium on board. Selenium levels below the RDA were associated in research with a failure to ovulate. In addition, plasma selenium levels help regulate estradiol levels throughout the menstrual cycle.[193]

Get Your Boron

Low brain activity is linked to reduced arousal. Good thing we have Boron, which improves cognitive function and optimizes our brain's electrical activity. It does other stuff, like grow bones and heal wounds, aids in absorbing magnesium and giving us antioxidant benefits.

But it wouldn't be in this list if it didn't play an important role in the regulation of sex hormones.[194] Increasing boron significantly raises testosterone and estradiol levels. Boron also has the effect of amplifying androgens, increasing their bioavailability. Leafy greens, legumes and nuts are wonderful sources of boron. (And taking boron will also help you remember that.)

Go Nuts for Mineral Balance

I mentioned supplementation in some studies, but eating our minerals is the best bet for avoiding any issues. Many minerals compete in our bodies, and without securing a clearly diagnosed deficiency, increasing one on the fly can trigger a deficiency in another.

For instance, research has demonstrated that high iron intake can inhibit zinc absorption,[195] and calcium can inhibit iron absorption. Likewise, taking too much magnesium can cause low calcium, which can be dangerous.

Enter: nuts. Like leafy greens, nuts contain loads of essential minerals, but more importantly, are already perfectly mineral balanced. Eating nuts reduces the risk of respiratory diseases, Type 2 diabetes,[196] cancer, cardiovascular disease and infections.[197] Nuts also improve gut microbial diversity,[198] which is associated with various measures of overall health.

Research bore this out: One study examined healthy males with satisfying sex lives. Half of the participants added about two handfuls of nuts daily, and both groups reported their results during the experiment. The group who added nuts to their diet significantly increased the intensity of orgasms as well as sexual desire.[199] In another study, pistachio nuts daily, specifically, improved all aspects of erectile function and increased penile blood flow and promoted better cholesterol levels. Come for the better cholesterol,[200] but stay for the better sex.

Or rather, let's save our experimentation for the bedroom, not our mineral balance. For the bedroom, I say go nuts.

Why Not Walnuts?

When it comes to walnuts, it's hard to argue with history. Humans have gathered and eaten walnuts since at least 7300 BCE and Greeks cultivated them as early as 4000 BCE. We've definitely been having sex ever since.

In traditional Chinese medicine, walnuts, which coincidentally resemble the human brain, have been considered a brain food for millennia. Walnuts contain ALA (alpha-linolenic acid), which, in research, improved how fast nerves fire in patients with nerve damage.[201]

All-a you need to know is that in addition to being great sources of ALA, walnuts contain l-arginine, the precursor of nitric oxide, which increases clitoral and penile blood flow and is essential to sexual pleasure.

Walnuts are also loaded with phenolic antioxidants, which protect the structure of arteries carrying blood to the genitals.[202] And it's another case where you can see results by popping a few before sex. One study demonstrated that, within four hours of eating walnuts, blood vessels are more elastic, which is, again, better for that blood flow. They also counteract bad food choices, offsetting the negative effects of a high-fat meal on your artery's walls.[203]

Dietary Nitrates

Nitrate-rich foods such as leafy greens, celery and beets reduce blood pressure and make the vascular system more pliable. The nitrates in these foods convert to nitric oxide (NO), which we know promotes vascular health. NO has anti-inflammatory properties and prevents blood clots. It also dilates blood vessels and makes them more elastic, delivering good blood supply to the penis, vagina and clitoris. Bonus: This is also a surefire way to enhance stamina because it improves delivery of oxygen to muscles, reducing fatigue.

To get more nitrates, instead of simply chowing down, a lot of studies have tried to see if nitrate supplements were as effective. Sorry to say, they found that these were detrimental to health. So, the healthiest way to increase nitric oxide is through dietary sources, not pills, a recurring theme here.

There are cases where some nitrates outshine their peers. Beets and spinach are like the Prom King and Queen of Nitrate High, showing stellar performance.[204] Like couples on prom night, they go to town immediately. Even after a single serving of spinach, the blood vessels become more elastic. In one study, salivary nitrate increased eightfold a mere two hours after eating spinach and blood vessels were measurably more elastic.[205]

So, if you and your partner are going to be getting busy, try spinach and beets a couple hours beforehand to enhance blood flow to the genitals, which will make for more pleasurable sex. If the thought of those super-foods leaves you wanting, there are plenty other choices.

Foods high in naturally-occurring nitrates[206]:

Moderate	High	Very High
Cabbage	Parsley	Beets
Turnips	Leeks	Celery
Dill	Swiss Chard	Green Lettuces
	Fennel	Radish
	Endive	Spinach

Because these high-nitrate foods have such an immediate benefit to blood vessels, they should be included in a date-night sex menu (see chapter 14 for a more detailed menu).

Improving the Flow of Qi and Blood for Great Sex

Science continually discovers evidence of what the Chinese understood in ancient times. Keeping the vessels unblocked allows for blood to flow freely to the sex organs. The food we eat strongly influences vascular health and its ability to deliver good blood supply.

The role of the blood is to nourish all of the tissues of the body, from our skin, hair and organs, to our penis, vagina and clitoris. This important role can either be enhanced or impeded by the food we eat. Potassium-rich foods, and those high in naturally-occurring nitrates, such as spinach, luxuriate the vessels, while fatty foods stiffen them. Nuts, especially walnuts, with their omega 3s, essential minerals and antioxidants, also promote vascular health and support great sex.

You can incorporate these dietary recommendations by getting into healthier habits. A great lunchtime routine is to have a big leafy green salad with walnuts and whatever vegetables you like, and add a baked potato, yam or squash. This is both a satisfying meal and a sex-healthy one.

While the qi, or nerve impulses, command the blood, the vessels carry the blood. When qi and blood flow freely through the vessels to our sex organs, we experience magnificent sexual pleasure and powerful orgasm.

PART II:
ANCIENT CHINESE
WISDOM FOR GREAT SEX

TRADITIONAL CHINESE MEDICINE PAST AND PRESENT

Simply put, the Chinese really knew how to get busy. I know what you're thinking: Doesn't the population itself worldwide prove that all cultures clearly have no trouble figuring out how to get it on? The answer is yes, but we aren't just talking about procreation here. And the ancient Chinese brought particular flair to the art of sex.

Free and Easy

Springtime in ancient China was once the season for sex. Nature set the scene, and nature was generous: Vibrant pink azaleas and peonies decorated the countryside, and sweet orchids perfumed the breeze. As the land's beautiful gifts emerged, people took time to celebrate their ripening bodies with erotic festivals.[207]

Women, the great initiators of sex and guardians of all sexual knowledge, prayed to the many gods (ahem, modern women are not so different). They prayed to the kitchen god, they prayed to the wealth god. They asked the god of joy for a good life, and to throw in a good husband while they were at it.

Each young man, the ignorant pupil in sex, the green dragon, hoped that one beautiful white tiger would open her mysterious gate and let him explore her jade hall.[208]

The entire community got in on this mating season. In houses surrounded by bamboo, obedient girls prepared for the festival with their mothers.

They may have cooked up an enormous feast of rice dumplings, millet wine, yellow rice and perhaps a nice rabbit with ginger and mushrooms or roasted duck with fennel, anise and black pepper.

As the grains matured, those hard-working men spent long, hot days in the fields, and a festival for sex seemed like a great idea to them, too. Clad in indigo-dyed hemp pants and jackets, they offered sacrifices to the ancestors to keep them happy and benevolent. If the ancestors were pleased, they brought peace and fortune, which explains why Chinese wanted to have many sons, as they could care for the ancestors with abundant sacrifices.

After all that hard work and prep by the entire community, it would be time for the men to make a difficult choice: which young lady with which to copulate after the roasted duck. He could only choose one to court and hook up with, but it wasn't a speedy race against time. Even as fall began and the fragrance of Osmanthus blossoms filled the air, he would continue to draw on her essences, the well that never ran dry. The spirit of the valley. They might even formalize their union before the coming of cold weather, especially if she got pregnant. But maybe not. Either of them could back out.

Royally Screwed

For nobility, on the other hand, there were greater gains but bigger sacrifices. Nobility knew the ancestors were already smiling down on them due to their vast power and wealth, but in return, the ancestors asked for a lot, requiring immense sacrifices to be made regularly by males of the family.

The male rulers, in their long silk patterned robes with flowing ribbons, possessed a great amount of power, or "de" from their ancestors. That meant an emperor's ancestors would require the grandest sacrifices of all to be kept happy. If they were displeased, they might turn wicked and bring disaster to him and his family. His utmost duty would be to produce copious male heirs to continue showering the ancestors in payment, and in order to produce plenty of male children, he was going to need a long list of willing female partners.

Here, an emperor could rack up the kind of partners fit for, well, a king. There was the queen or empress, of course, but she only put out on a full moon, as that was believed to be the best time to conceive. For the rest, she outsourced that endless work to lower-ranking ladies (lucky girls), so that he'd have three consorts, nine second rank wives, twenty-seven third rank wives, and eighty-one concubines (notice that they are all multiples of three, by intent).

No way could he keep all their names straight, which is why he kept a tablet of his faves, the original little black book. Probably best not to remember all their names, anyway. Rulers were known to have as many as 3,000 lonely concubines, and it would be impossible to field that many complaints on the job.

Unbelievably, there was actually enough time left over for other types of fun, and emperors could and did also have dalliances with men. Though male homosexuality was considered immoral later on, it was popular in the Song, Ming and Qing dynasties. Emperors in the Han dynasty were recorded to have male sexual subordinates.

By now you've got to be wondering how on earth any of these women or men knew what day was their sex day with the big guy. Obviously, they had a sex calendar. It was a big job and a big deal, handled by a sex secretary (sex *administrative assistant*) or lady of the court, who jotted down the hundreds of sex staffers' go-times in vermillion ink, made of cinnabar. It was coded, too! Each rank had a specific frequency of sex on specific days. For instance, on nine days of the month the guy entertained groups of nine concubines, then the other assorted sex people had their days.

There was a reason that concubines did all the heavy lifting: The emperor was supposed to copulate with them more than the higher-ranking women to nourish his sex essence and increase the possibility of an heir by having as many children as possible.

While all sex is considered an exchange of yin and yang, there was a particular focus on what female sexuality gave in energy to a powerful male. Woman's vaginal secretions contained precious jing, the vital essence of life. Woman produced jing, and man absorbed it, extending his life and strengthening his vital force.

So an emperor would build up his potency with the lowly women to boost up the quality of sperm he in turn served to the empress. Now that's a community effort. That concubine-infused emperor sperm would then help prime the empress for creating the strongest, healthiest and most intelligent heir to the throne possible.

Though this seems all too convenient to be granted moral sanction to regularly have sex with 120 women outside ones marriage, they did it for their country and their heirs. Heroes selflessly doing what was best for baby. It's no surprise, though, that if you were a male commoner in that system, you could not go around impregnating as many women as you wanted. Fittingly, the punishment for male commoner promiscuity was castration.

Imperial women had their fun too. They might also have a harem of men, and there are records of one princess having sexual encounters with thirty men at once (damn, girl).[209] Female homosexuality was tolerated in earlier times, especially for the lonely concubines, who finally get a break here, as they're not allowed to sleep with other men.

And they could have a lot more fun with women: Ancient sex toys have been identified, including ribbed, double-ended dildos carved out of ivory or other materials. They would have silk belts tied to both sides so that both women could be pleasured at the same time. They also used herbs such as Suo Yang, which they would insert into their vagina. This herb would expand by absorbing vaginal secretions — nature's penis.

Let's Talk About Sex

You gotta hand it to imperial physicians and advisors. They were prolific writers and produced numerous sex manuals in ancient times for our enjoyment today. Here men and women were told exactly what to do to keep the empire's sexual ecosystem up and running.

Man, the leader of the family, was instructed something we're just now getting around to telling modern men today: that he should learn how to please all of his wives, consorts and concubines, making them orgasm with every intercourse. Every. Single. One.

Obviously, this was an easy idea to sell when it contributed to the community goal of making more and better children. Su Nu, female advisor to the "Yellow Emperor," described ways to identify sexual satisfaction in women for this very purpose. A satisfied woman would produce the most jing, or vital essence, which the man would absorb, promoting vitality and longevity.

It was also considered a moral duty to follow the prescribed schedule of sex with all of their wives and assorted sex personnel. Ancient texts explained that it was depressing for the poor, lonely house servant and concubine who was not tended to sexually, and no one wants a depressed woman producing bummed-out heirs.

Some of the texts were helpfully specific. One recounts forty-three styles of sex practiced by an imperial official with his consort in gardens and in the woods. The mind reels, but again, the goal is logistical: In pleasing so many women, rulers had to maintain optimal sexual health to ensure that they cared for both their lovers and their heirs.

Just Don't Blow Your Load

The above would have you believe that nothing was better for ancient China than constant, varied sex with as many partners, in as many positions, and as many settings as is humanly possible in a calendar day. However, with different dynasties came different beliefs.

Though sex was long thought to be nourishing, the Chinese grew to believe that ejaculating too frequently would deplete man's vital life essence and were thus encouraged to orgasm without ejaculating (no easy feat). More contemporary traditional Chinese physicians are in line with this and have written countless case studies of male patients suffering illness or death due to excessive masturbation.

The notion of restraint here was that if sperm was conserved, it could travel along the spine to the brain and then to the Sea of Qi, bathing the body and mind in luxurious essence. The woman's essence was thought to *only* be nourished by sex and orgasm, which must be why women were always trying to entice men into the act, or so they believed.

Traditional Chinese views on sexuality were not always so buttoned up. Before Taoism (600 BC) this concept didn't exist, while later Confucianist proscriptions were more repressive. These were times of great political upheaval, with dynasties struggling to maintain power through control of its citizens. Philosophy was very much interwoven with government, and these belief systems grew in a time of increasing government control in Chinese life.

Uniformity in Confucius philosophy was required, and rulers used Confucianism as a tool of state control, even when it came to how its private citizens engaged in sex. Deviation from prescribed standards of behavior and acting instead on one's own accord were tantamount to treason. There were severe penalties for deviating from prescribed sexual standards.

It may not be coincidence then that the medical views of sexual temperance and sexual repression coincided with these socio-political ideologies. Nevertheless, it is still a part of traditional Chinese medicine practiced today. In aiming for proper sexual function, modern texts advise avoiding excessive masturbation and obscene visual stimulation. Here, too much of a good thing quickly becomes a bad thing.

Not Too Hot, Not Too Cold

There is, then, too much sex. But there is also too little.

Some physicians have written in ancient texts about sexual frustration causing disease. Qi (pronounced "chi" or "chee") is the vital life force that courses through our bodies. Unattended arousal and loneliness inhibited the free flow of qi, causing depression.[210] According to one ancient physician, when the mind longs for sexual pleasure, and the body is denied, it causes stagnation in the heart and mind.

We don't need medicine to tell us that human beings innately long for warmth, affection and love from a sexual partner, though ancient physicians took note of this. They believed the lack of sex diminished health and caused disease, so sexual activity was necessary for good health in men and women.

Other texts discussed sexual intercourse as a spiritual practice which brought greater health benefits with more abundant sex. More sex would generate more jing, which would replenish life force and promote longevity. In addition, there are Taoist texts that describe special sexual positions which cure or prevent illness.

What Say You, Traditional Chinese Medicine?

TCM tells us that yin and yang are the way of life, the way of sex, the way of heaven and of earth. Heaven and earth were separated in humans who suffer an eternal death as a result. We defy death in sex, as yin and yang are reunited.

Yin is intuitive. She slinks through the cold dark night, illuminated by the moonlight. Yang is a force to be reckoned with. He gallops through the heavens, worshipping the sun. Sex is a merging of yin and yang essences, of heaven and earth. The feminine yin sexual energy and the masculine yang energy combine and nurture each other. Water cools the scorching fire and, in doing so, is warmed by its heat.

Yin and yang, being inseparable and rooted in each other, are both needed in abundance for great sex. Yin is the blood and the fluids, while yang is the nerve impulse and muscle contraction. The yang squeezes the blood vessels, propelling the yin blood through the arteries and to the genitals. The yang qi contains the yin blood in the vessels. Conversely, qi engenders blood. The hot yang excites our sexual passions, and the yin blood fills the sex organs.

The essence of the body is housed in the kidneys. From this essence, life is possible, and when our essence runs out, life ceases. Male essence is embodied in sperm, and female essence is embodied in menses. The pre-heaven essence is what we are born with. It is the DNA in our genes, and it is the microbiome passed to us from our mother's birth canal and from her kisses. The post-heaven essence is what our body makes out of the food we eat.

Qi and Blood

As I've noted throughout the book, qi must flow freely for good health. Blockage or deficiency equals disease. In TCM, this is true throughout the body: it's the life force that courses through us, allows air to enter our lungs, and for the heart to contract. Qi moves food through us, from mouth to anus, via the digestive tract.

In sex, as you know now, qi is what drives blood to the genitals and keeps it there. The vessels through which qi and blood flow can be understood as the nervous and vascular systems. When the vessels are blocked, as in the case with plaque accumulation, sexual function declines. Or when the qi is insufficient to conduct strong reliable nerve signals, pleasure decreases and less blood is directed to the penis or clitoris.

The function of blood is to nourish all the tissues in the entire body.[211] The heart governs the blood. Like yin and yang, qi and blood are mutually dependent. Qi commands the blood. The blood obeys the qi. Or translated into biomedicine: the nerve impulses (qi) command the blood (yin) to flow to the sex organs when we are aroused.

Qi is made by the power of digestion in our body. *Qi Hua* is the transformation of the food we eat into vital life force. This transformational function is attributed to the spleen qi in TCM. Spleen qi can be equated in many ways with the microbiome of the digestive tract.

When the spleen qi is strong, it is able to fully transform food and drink into the vital clear essence that nourishes the body and becomes qi to then be distributed throughout the body, and to the penis, vagina and clitoris. This force courses through the vessels and nerves, sending sizzling vitality to the sex organs.

Just a Little Prick

Diet is the fuel we need for great sex, and our body is the car that drives the passion. Acupuncture, then, can be thought of as the toolkit that fine tunes our bodies to keep them functioning optimally.

But what, exactly, is acupuncture and how does it do this?

Acupuncture is a system of medicine used to treat various physical, mental and emotional conditions and to alleviate pain. It works by strengthening the physical condition and harmonizing the body systems to promote longevity and healing.

Understood traditionally, acupuncture works by circulating qi, or vital life force, throughout the vessels of the body. From a biomedical perspective, acupuncture improves microcirculation, regulates the body's respiration, temperature, blood pressure, hormonal secretion and immune response. It also stimulates the central nervous system and affects the release of basic body chemicals, called neurotransmitters, throughout the body.

Originating in ancient China, acupuncture is now widely practiced in the West. There is a growing body of research demonstrating the efficacy of acupuncture. For this reason, it is recognized as an effective therapy by the National Institute of Health and the World Health Organization.

How is it performed? By inserting fine needles into various points on the body, anywhere from millimeters (on hands and feet, for example) to several inches (hips, for example) into the body. I've discussed meridians or pathways already in the book, and the body contains twelve regular meridians, with hundreds of acupuncture points.

When treating a patient, I first assess the relative status of qi and blood, yin and yang. I also note dysfunction of bodily organs as understood by traditional Chinese medicine. Locations for needle insertions are selected to harmonize imbalances. The patient's treatment plan is designed based on their diagnosis and symptoms.

About those needles: I understand that many people are needle-squeamish, but there's no need for that with acupuncture. For starters, it's important to realize that acupuncture is a pain relief treatment too. Studies have shown that acupuncture can moderate dopamine in the body, making patients feel less pain and an increased sense of well-being.

Acupuncture needles are also very fine. They're so fine in fact that about 40 of them could fit into the barrel of a hypodermic needle. This means they're generally quite comfortable, and any sensation felt will be like a very mild prick—not close to the sensation of getting a shot.

For treating sexual function specifically, needle placement often includes the perineum, the fleshy area between the anus and testicles or vagina, which is a major crossing point of nerves associated with sexual function. However, in treating any condition, needles are placed both for symptoms and for the patient's unique constitution. For example, when I see patients looking to improve erectile strength, I might needle their perineum and also include points to harmonize the liver and spleen.

Once needles are placed, patients continue to lie on a massage table relaxing while listening to spa music. Treatment sessions last about an hour, and most patients notice changes within a few treatments. A standard course of treatment is ten sessions but is highly variable.

As Chinese medicine and acupuncture are a holistic approach, no two people are the same, and every treatment is tailored to that person as a unique individual.

Overall, acupuncture is a treatment that leaves patients feeling good, which is exactly the mindset we seek for great sex.

TRADITIONAL CHINESE DIETETICS

Ancient Chinese physicians, such as the famous Sun Si-miao, recommended using diet as the very first approach in internal medicine. A well-balanced sex diet cares for the kidneys, which are the root of the essence. It also cares for the physical manifestation of essence, semen and menses. Such a diet luxuriates the vessels, allowing for the abundant free flow of qi and blood throughout the body. Great sex is a balance between yin, bodily substance and yang, bodily function.

In traditional Chinese dietetics, what a person should eat strongly depends on constitution. A true TCM dietary prescription would assess the individual person and make recommendations according to the individual's unique nature.

However, there are still some basic tenants of healthy eating, and some specific to good sexual function, we can generally and safely apply from TCM guidance.

Overall, that's fresh foods, cooked and eaten within twenty-four hours of preparation. Longer periods will damage the qi of the food and engender damp. Traditional Buddhists encouraged eating vegetables over grains, which can lead to accumulation in the vessels.

While we each tend toward different imbalances, below are some common constitutions and general dietary guidelines to keep in mind. There are numerous other constitutions, and for a specific diagnosis, see your friendly neighborhood acupuncturist.

Blood/Yin Deficient

Blood deficiency is characterized by a dull, pale complexion, floaters in the eyes and muscle cramping. Someone who is yin deficient is typically a lanky person who might have difficulty putting weight on, for example, and can tolerate greater amounts of yin supplementing foods without as much concern over their cloying effect.

Foods to Limit: They should be mindful of drying or spicy hot foods that can further tax the yin.

Foods to Incorporate: Fats, nuts and oils.

Qi/Yang Deficient

Qi deficiency (a milder condition) and yang deficiency (a more severe condition) presents as patients who are cold and tired.

Foods to Limit: These people should especially avoid cold and raw foods, as they further damage the qi and deplete the yang.

Foods to Incorporate: Those who tend to feel cold should eat warm. When we say warming, we are referring to both the energetic properties of the food and the temperature. That is, the *temperature* heat and the *spice* heat. Warm foods include obvious foods such as soups, stews, and porridge, but also spices such as cinnamon, fennel, cloves and black pepper.

Stagnation of Damp, Phlegm and Blood

A damp constitution is someone who tends toward heaviness and is easily phlegmy, sinusy, and congested, someone with plaque accumulation or who retains water.

Foods to Limit: Avoid rich, cloying foods, as they will contribute to this stagnation in the body. This blockage restricts the free flow of qi and blood. Cloying foods include rich, greasy and excessively sweet foods such as dairy, sweet drinks, fatty meats and baked goods. This constitution should also avoid cold and raw foods.

Foods to Incorporate: Since phlegm always arises from a weak spleen qi, the spleen must be strengthened with the foods we eat (see above).

Acrid flavors like ginger, garlic, leeks, cardamom and cherries are good for those who have cold phlegm, and bitter cool flavors like green leaves such as dandelion or endive for those with heat phlegm. Also good for heat phlegm are mung beans, pears, grapes, algae like seaweed, carp and radish.[212] Consult a practitioner for a specific diagnosis.

Cloying Foods Are Bad News

A general note: For abundant qi and blood flowing to the genitals, we should *all* avoid cloying foods no matter our constitution. Phlegm blockage and water retention are very common with the standard American diet, which is high in sugar, salt and fat and can be understood as anything that blocks the vessels. Drinking too much booze also generates more phlegm and excessive heat.

Flavor, Temperature

As I've mentioned, there are five flavors we must happily balance for an ideal sex diet: sweet, salty, bitter, sour and acrid (aka pungent or spicy). Foods are classified in TCM according to flavor and energetic temperature and also according to the organs they influence. Energetically hot foods like lamb, salmon, cinnamon, garlic, and ginger warm the yang. Cold foods like mung beans, melons, cucumber and salads nourish the cool yin.

Pathogens are called evils in Chinese medicine and may include heat, cold, damp, wind and dryness. These evils may loosely correspond to different microbes. Heat often corresponds to bacteria, cold to viruses and damp to fungus. In Chinese herbal medicine, as in dietary therapy, we use cold to combat heat and heat to combat cold.

For example, strep throat is a heat condition. As such, we use very cold herbs in treatment. However, we must be cautious because too much cold can damage the spleen qi (microbiome). Over time, our diet determines our microbial populations, as has been documented in research.

The energetic temperature of foods relates to the degree to which it has either a warming or cooling effect on the body. Hot and warm foods are yang in nature, and cool and cold foods are yin in nature. Temperature and flavor must be balanced in the diet, especially in accordance with one's constitution.

Sweet

Sweet is the flavor of the earth, corresponding to the spleen. It's also the flavor winner for easiest to overeat because most foods have sweet in their flavor profile. This would include foods that we don't necessarily think of as being sweet, such as rice and oats, as well as apples, spinach, chicken, almonds and pumpkin.

Sweet foods nourish the qi and blood, but in excess, can be cloying. In contrast, foods which are light and airy nourish the body without creating blockage of qi.

Salty

The salty flavor corresponds to the kidneys and to water. It is a yin flavor which cools, moistens and softens. It's also the other flavor we're most likely to overeat, giving sweet a run for its money.

Naturally, energetically "salty" foods include meat and fish, seaweed and need not include added salt to be balanced. But as salt dehydrates the body and damages the yin fluid, blood and vessels of the body, most of us should be looking to reduce our intake and shift it toward the above options.

Bitter

Bitter is the flavor of the heart and corresponds to fire. And as you might guess, it's the flavor most sorely lacking in our diet.

Bitter foods, namely vegetables and including leafy greens such as spinach, kale, romaine, green leaf lettuces, parsley, cilantro and other greens, accomplish a great deal in the body and get a bad rep all for not being sweet.

But they're magic in our bodies. First, the bitter flavor clears heat and drains damp. It can also buffer the other cloying foods in our diet that generate dampness.

During the hot yang summer, or when we are feeling stressed or overly excited with joy, we should turn to bitter foods, as this is the flavor of the heart. Too much bitter, however, can have a laxative effect.

Sour

Sour is the flavor of the liver and gallbladder and corresponds to wood. It astringes fluids and supplements yin.

So why are we so sour about it? We should focus on this flavor in the springtime, or when we are irritable or angry, as this is the emotion of the liver. Sour foods include apples, oranges, mangoes, lemons, limes and most other fruits.

Acrid (Pungent or Spicy)

Acrid is the flavor corresponding to the lungs and metal. Acrid flavor moves qi, promotes circulation and disperses stagnation.

It's found in many culinary herbs and spices, including thyme, cinnamon, garlic and ginger. Other acrid foods include onions, chili peppers, radishes and watercress. Acrid flavors are beneficial in the colder months and when we are experiencing sadness. However, eating too many acrid and spicy foods is inadvisable because it can generate heat.

Cold

According to traditional Chinese medicine, eating physically cold (iced coffee) or energetically cold foods (dairy) can damage the spleen qi. It can also injure kidney qi and kidney yang, which fuel the ministerial fire of libido. Cold food causes stagnation and especially should not be eaten frozen, such as in frozen smoothies. Excessively sweet and fatty ice cream would be particularly insulting to the spleen qi because it is cloying, rich and also cold in temperature.

A discrepancy exists between modern research and traditional Chinese dietary principles when it comes to salad. TCM advises against eating raw foods including salad, preferring to instead cook leafy greens. Research overwhelmingly favors abundant consumption of salads and raw vegetables in general, demonstrating that they have the highest vitamin content compared with cooked vegetables. TCM argues that, while raw produce may have higher vitamin content, the vitamins from cooked foods are more assimilable and therefore healthier.

One cooking method that is highly recommended in TCM is slow, long cooking, which nourishes the spleen qi. This would include congee, which is a thick grain porridge, such as oats or rice cooked in a crock pot with fruits and/or vegetables and perhaps a small amount of beans, meat or fish. This type of meal is often served to people when they are ill. Soups and stews that are light in fat content would also be beneficial.

A Meaty Moment

In traditional Chinese medicine, avoiding meat is not recommended. According to TCM, meat is a blood tonic and lack thereof will cause blood deficiency. Having said that, people in ancient China would not have eaten the huge quantities that we do today in the US. They would have eaten mostly rice, vegetables and sometimes a small amount of meat.

Nobility, who did indulge in more meat, tended toward obesity and conditions such as gout. Pork is the most dampening or cloying, followed by beef. Modern research supports the traditional Chinese view that excessive meat consumption blocks the vessels, due to its high fat content. This fat blocks arteries in the tendon of the liver (the penis), as well as the vagina and clitoris, causing reduced sexual pleasure and function for males and females.

Blood deficiency is consistent with conditions like anemia and B-12 deficiency. Vegans can supplement B-12 to ensure their bodies are getting sufficient quantities. Vegetarians can obtain it from eggs. Taking iron without a diagnosed deficiency is inadvisable.

Diet and Libido

Sex drive comes from the ministerial fire between our kidneys and depends on adequate kidney qi and kidney yang. Conversely, when kidney yin is deficient, this causes high libido without satisfaction in sex. For great sex, the foods we eat must nourish the kidneys. Times have changed though. You can't just munch on a seal or tiger penis to boost your game in the bedroom. Or can you? In fact, there are restaurants in China, who, rather than Peking Duck, serve up dishes of bull, seal and snake dicks. No tigers though, as its illegal, but is purchased on the black market. For those of us who care about these animals, we can increase libido and sexual function by eating the following foods instead:

Foods to Warm and Nourish Kidney Qi and Yang

These foods should be prepared using warming cooking methods such as boiling, grilling and pan frying.

- Meat: Venison, poultry, lamb, gecko, goat, duck, human placenta
- Fish: Eel, shrimp, oysters, mussels
- Fruit: Raisins, cherries, raspberries
- Vegetables: Fennel, leeks, yams, sea cucumber
- Grains: Oats, corn
- Legumes: Lentils, kidney beans, black beans
- Nuts/Seeds: Chestnuts, pistachios, walnuts

The following culinary herbs boost sexual function and libido by nourishing kidney yang or promoting the circulation of qi and blood[213]:

Rosemary: Warm, bitter and acrid, rosemary warms and nourishes kidney qi and yang.

Star Anise (Da Hui Xiang): Sweet, warm and acrid, star anise warms and nourishes kidney qi and yang.

Garlic (Da Suan): Warm and acrid garlic warms digestive function, and promotes the circulation of qi and blood.

Ginger (Jiang): Hot, acrid ginger warms the digestive function and promotes the circulation of qi and blood.

Fenugreek seeds (Hu Lu Ba): Warm and bitter fenugreek nourishes kidney yang and disperses damp-cold.

Cinnamon (Rou Gui): Warm to hot in nature, cinnamon warms the digestive function and promotes circulation of qi and blood. It also warms kidney yang, activates blood circulation and expels internal cold.

Clove (Ding Xiang): Warm and spicy, cloves warm the digestive function and kidney yang.

Black cardamom: (Yi Zhi Ren): Warm and acrid black cardamom warms kidney yang and secures the essence

Foods to Enhance Sexual Function by Nourishing Kidney Yin

Black sesame seeds (Hei Zhi Ma): Sweet and neutral black sesame seeds tonify kidney yin

Asparagus tuber (Tian Men Dong): Sweet, bitter and very cold asparagus tuber nourishes kidney yin.

Wood Ear mushroom (Yin Er): Sweet in flavor, it promotes the movement of qi and blood, and removes stagnation. Tastes great in a soup. Traditionally it is not known to enter the kidney channel, but modern research has demonstrated its aphrodisiac properties, as noted in chapter 13.

Goji berries (Gou Qi Zi): Sweet and neutral goji berries nourish kidney yin and mildly tonify kidney yang

Chinese Medicinal Herbs

If you go to a traditional Chinese herbalist, he or she may prescribe some of the following herbs for enhancing sexual function in both men and women. Medicinal herbs should not be self-prescribed though. While they often have a more gentle action than pharmaceuticals, they may have quite a strong biological action on the body. In fact, the biologically active components of most pharmaceuticals today were originally identified in plants and fungus. (For instance, Artemesia annua, used since ancient times to treat malaria in traditional Chinese medicine, was developed into an effective pharmaceutical treatment).

The bottom line is that herbs are drugs and should be prescribed by someone who understands the pharmacokinetics of herbs, dosage and how to modify herbs based on your response to treatment. Anyone considering traditional Chinese herbal medicine should consult a trained professional. Practitioners of traditional Chinese medicine generally have a master's degree in herbal medicine. He or she will prescribe an herbal formula that is right for the patient's constitution and presenting concerns. A more detailed description of many of these medicinals appears in Chapter 13, Aphrodisiacs.

Herbs to Nourish Kidney Qi, Yang for Libido, Sexual Function

- Cordyceps
- Eucommia
- Astragalus seeds
- Ginseng
- Morinda root
- Psoralea fruit
- Deer velvet
- Deer antler gelatin
- Deer antler
- Cistanche
- Cynomorii stem
- Cuscuta
- Curculigo
- Epimedium
- Chinese raspberry
- Snidium seed
- Cornus

Herbs to Nourish Kidney Yin:

- American ginseng
- Cooked rehmannia root
- Lily bulb
- Fresh water turtle plastron
- Turtle shell gelatin
- Ophiopogon tuber
- Herba Ecliptae
- Ligustrum
- Dendrobium

Again, consult a professional licensed practitioner of traditional Chinese herbal medicine for a proper herbal prescription.

Summary of Traditional Chinese Dietary Recommendations for Great Sex

The art of sex, or merging of yin and yang, is cultivated by thoughtfully caring for one's body. A body that is well nourished will allow for the free flow of life's vital substances, qi, blood and jing. The vessels that carry the essences of sex must be cared for by eating a balanced diet where each of the five flavors is represented. In addition, we must avoid rich, greasy and processed foods that block the vessels.

Eating fresh, cooked foods and avoiding cold raw foods will be best for the spleen which generates qi and blood. For boosting sexual fitness, eat foods and spices that nourish the kidneys, which are the root of the essence. Through this thoughtful self-care, we can strengthen our vital force, as we awaken from death, reuniting heaven and earth.

PART III:
ENVIRONMENT AND
LIFESTYLE FOR GREAT SEX

Great Sex is in the Living and Breathing

José came home sweating from his run. *Working out always makes me horny,* he thought when he saw his boyfriend Robert sitting on the couch glued to his iPhone as usual. He walked over and playfully straddled him, positioning his crotch directly at Robert's eye level, and unzipped his own pants, hoping Robert would take the not-so-subtle hint.

Nothing. Robert eyes were still on his phone. He had gotten an annoying email from a co-worker and was not in the mood.

After dinner, José tried again. This time, he put his hand on Robert's ass and squeezed firmly, something that had always worked to lighten things up when they were first dating. Unmoved, Robert kept scrolling on Instagram. He lit up a cigarette and continued to check his likes.

At bedtime, José went in for a third attempt to connect with Robert. He decided to wait up for him in bed, naked and rock hard. Surely then he'd notice how much José wanted him. Instead, Robert barely glanced his way, tossing his phone on the night stand and opening his laptop. He was tired and wanted to stream his favorite show.

José finally spoke up. He told Robert that he didn't feel cared for in the relationship. He wanted to connect with him physically and sexually, but Robert was always distracted. It was bad enough that they hadn't had a conversation all day, let alone watching Robert sit around all the time on his phone.

Robert, for his part, thought that their sex life was just fine. They did it about as much as any other couple that had been together for four years.

Work was stressful, and he felt that he took on a lot of responsibility, while José had a carefree job as a graphic artist. Robert didn't even have time to do the things he enjoyed in life, like hiking and riding his bike, let alone sex. He loved José but didn't understand why he couldn't just jerk off if he was that horny and respect that Robert was stressed out and tired.

José took Robert's phone and showed him that his daily screen time was over four hours. Robert realized that, while he never seemed to have time to do anything he enjoyed, he always had hours to spend on his phone, which was an escape and not a solution. Both wanted to try to save their relationship and were willing to make changes. He decided that it was time to focus back in on their connection rather than take it for granted. José agreed to take more responsibility to ease some of Robert's stress.

Together, José and Robert developed a few new daily habits. After a healthy dinner, they would take a walk around the local park, and on Saturdays they hiked or biked.

I treated Robert with acupuncture to quit smoking, and soon he noticed he had much more energy. Even better, he always seemed to be in the mood for sex after a hike, instead of tired and ready to zone out.

José and Robert's relationship is strikingly common. Though we've no doubt heard a million warnings about screen time, the truth is, our modern way of life puts pressure on us to spend hours a day on our phones and little to no time being physically active. This is contrary to the biological design of human beings. Our qi and blood are meant to move. Exercise facilitates the movement of the vital essences of sex.

Exercise is much more than a component of good health, and it's not just a means to an end to look good. It's as essential for great sex as the food we eat.

Add to this the significant amount of environmental pollutants we absorb daily from industrial waste and electromagnetic fields—another assault on a great sex life—and most of us are struggling to offset lifestyle and environment that thwarts even the best efforts to optimize sexual health.

For these, TCM also offers essential guidance.

Exercise

At this point in history, talking at you about the numerous, life-changing benefits of exercise is about like hearing "Stairway to Heaven" in a guitar store. We are so super-saturated with this fact that our brains have become inured to it.

We get it. It's great for us. We should all do it, a lot more. We don't do it enough, and it's killing us.

It's been difficult for modern medicine to find a way to connect exercise to our everyday existence, or rather, to help us truly make the connection that physical movement, or lack thereof, is directly connected to how we feel every minute of every day. Our physical state affects how we experience life when we first wake up, as we sustain ourselves through work, childcare, relationships and socializing, and even when we sleep, how well we sleep, and also, of course, how we age. It affects mood, appetite, self-esteem, cognitive function. There is no part of every waking and sleeping moment of our lives that is not tied to our body's level of fitness in some way or another.

But enough about that. Let's make this about sex!

Exercise fuels better sex in every way. It's not just endurance, or stamina, but responsiveness, energy and lightness. It does this through impacting sex-related hormones such as estrogen, prolactin, cortisol, oxytocin and testosterone. It increases libido in humans across the board. For males, getting your body moving improves erectile function[214] and heightens sexuality. For females, it facilitates arousal and produces the kind of orgasms you want to tell your friends about. Even small bouts of exercise drastically improve sexual function.

Some research suggests we can predict sexual satisfaction by percentage of body fat. More body fat is associated with greater sexual dysfunction in males and females. Moving our bodies helps balance our weight and reduce body fat. According to research, exercise enhances cardiovascular endurance, which increases positive female sexual behavior.[215] In males, aerobic exercise done about three times a week for an hour led to more sex, more satisfying orgasms and better sexual function.[216]

Under forty? A study[217] found that men who exercise in their thirties have better erectile function. Even for those who already had erectile issues, forty minutes of moderate exercise four times a week helped. Because exercising essentially improves underlying issues of weight, hypertension, metabolic syndrome and cardiovascular disease, erections became stronger and easier to achieve after just spending some time moving around.[218]

Research has also found a connection[219] between how much we move and how much we get turned on, and get off. Females who exercise regularly have a much easier time becoming aroused and have more satisfying orgasms. Frequent exercisers among males have better erectile function. Other studies find that females who exercise prior to sexual stimuli become more easily aroused when exposed to them.[220] This is because stimulation of the sympathetic nervous system, which happens with exercise, also facilitates physical sexual response.

It's also a gut thing. The human microbiome, which affects nearly all aspects of our health, is positively altered through movement. It increases microbial diversity, reduces populations of microbes associates with disease and increases populations associated with health.[221]

I understand that many of us are exercise-averse, whether because of our schedules, free time, commitments or simply personal preferences. For every person who makes it seem effortless to habitually hit the gym (it's okay to loathe them), others among us find that the two hours required to travel, get dressed, hit the locker room and all the back and forth make a forty-five minute workout far too much of a hassle to keep it up.

But if you were to just see China on any given morning, where people gather in parks and in public spaces, young and old, all doing tai qi—a series of slow, meditative movements—in unison, I think you would start to approach exercise differently from the hurried, Western way we see it.

This is a fun way for people to come together, organic to their daily schedule, and a surprisingly good workout. Best of all, it doesn't feel like some huge identity shift, but rather, finding space within our days to incorporate into the world we inhabit. We don't need to kill it with a celebrity-worthy workout schedule to achieve general fitness either. We can aim for something that fits naturally within our own environments and lives, as well as our schedules.

To do this, I inventory my patients' exercise habits, daily schedules and various aversions to find ways to incorporate exercise into their daily routine at work and home, without requiring arduous alterations.

Taking thirty minutes of your lunch or break time to take a turn around the building, or a walk outdoors, is one such way. Many of us have jobs which are mentally fatiguing. Sometimes taking even just a few minutes when we are busy with projects at work will help to reset our concentration and mental energy. The reward is greater productivity in turn, which recuperates the time.

Also, some find it helpful to use the stairs in their own houses during the cold months. When it's warm, you can bike to the store instead of driving. In parking lots, park farther away to build in more steps for the trip. Building a consistent routine is most effective, and even small amounts offer great short- and long-term benefits.

José and Robert found ways to both get more exercise and spend time together all at once. This improved their connection and also improved their sexual health. Robert had more energy and higher libido, and both had improved arousal.

Sleep

Sleep is important for countless processes in the body, and lack of it can cause system-wide disruption. In TCM, it's where yang meets yin and transitions into restorative and calming sleep. Adequate sleep is not just necessary for work, and childcare, and exercise, and life. It's essential for great sex.

Dopamine is irreplaceable in sexual arousal and performance. Sleep keeps dopamine levels stable, and lack of sleep disrupts them. When we don't get enough sleep, it also triggers an inflammatory cascade with vascular changes that impair blood vessels, keeping them from dilating and contracting appropriately.[222] Inflammation is one major culprit in sexual dysfunction. But in addition to the many health benefits of adequate sleep, many couples who have less sex complain that they are too tired.

Of course, everything here is interconnected. We get better sleep when we eat well and move our bodies, giving us critical energy for sex.

Mind, Spirit and Body

We can't control everything. Unless you can find an unpopulated corner of the globe to buffer against the environmental hazards of phones, computers and pollution, they'll find you.

There will always be a co-worker who raises our stress, there will always be responsibilities at home. But there can be peace in surrendering ourselves to this certainty. And our state of mind has a very real effect on the health of our bodies.

Toward that end, there are a number of practices that aid in connecting mind, spirit and body toward that peaceful acceptance.

Mindfulness practices are a kind of meditation in the moment that focuses our awareness on the present for small periods of time. In research[223] this has demonstrated the ability to reduce symptoms of anxiety and depression. One study,[224] for example, found that tai qi with mental imagery improved nerve conduction velocity in patients with Type 2 diabetes. Tai qi has benefit to our peace of mind, and depending on the routine, may benefit the body, as it provides strengthening movement.

Yoga is an exercise for both the body and the mind. It contributes to overall well-being and improved psychological, physical and emotional health. Furthermore, it has been shown in research[225] to improve female sexual health by increasing desire, arousal, lubrication, orgasm, satisfaction and reducing pain.

In my practice, we discuss the many ways to be mindful, including yoga, tai qi, breathing exercises, qi gong, meditation or walking in the woods. Find the way that works for you.

While the pressures of modern life make it difficult to have a sex-healthy lifestyle, there are lots of simple ways to nourish great sex. We can sleep adequately and find ways to incorporate exercise into our work and home routines. When we kindly care for our body, spirit and mind, sexuality will be divine.

HEAVY METAL EXPOSURE

I'm not talking about getting busy at a Metallica concert, unfortunately. Most people don't realize that we are exposed to a growing quantity of heavy metals in air, water, food and in our houses. Certain metal ions are essential for the human body but in excess can be quite toxic to our reproductive system.

A big one I mentioned before is cadmium, which contributes to chronic disease and in high doses can cause death. Cadmium is mined and then released into the air during smelting. In addition, industrial,[226] agricultural and sewage waste also contributes, as it easily accumulates in soil and agriculture. As a result, the food we eat is one of the biggest contributors of cadmium in our bodies. Cigarette smoke (first and secondhand) is another major contributor to cadmium exposure.

Poisoning by heavy metals is a common health problem due to all this industrial waste. There are certain illnesses that have been on the rise as a result, such as asthma. The prevalence of allergic/asthmatic diseases globally has increased steadily, now affecting about 30–40% of the world population.[227]

Heavy metals are known neurotoxins, genotoxins and carcinogens, which can lead to chronic disease and hinder recovery from illness. Research has shown that environmental exposure to lead, mercury, cadmium, copper, arsenic and nickel causes significant structural and functional disruptions in the endocrine system, affecting the adrenals, thyroid, testis, ovary and pancreas.

In men and women these toxic heavy metals also affect sex hormones, thyroid hormones and can cause Type 2 diabetes as well as testicular and ovarian injury, reducing reproductive performance.[228]

The Environmental Burden of Disease project[229] was launched by the World Health Organization to assess the impact of a slew of substances such as benzene, dioxins, secondhand smoke, formaldehyde, lead, traffic noise, ozone, particulate matter (PM2.5) and radon on human health in six countries (Belgium, Finland, France, Germany, Italy and the Netherlands). Scientists concluded that 3-7% of the burden of disease (that is, illness) in these countries is attributable to these nine environmental pollutants.

Airborne particulate matter was the leading risk factor, and some 112,000 years of healthy life per million people were lost due to exposure to these toxins. Considering how many other major factors impact health, like diet, lifestyle and exercise, this figure is remarkable.

Simply put, our organs can't handle it. The systems most commonly affected by heavy metal exposure include the central nervous system, gastrointestinal (GI) tract, cardiovascular system, hematopoietic (the production of blood cells and platelets within bones), renal and peripheral nervous systems.

By now, you'll have put together that these systems all very much affect sexual function and pleasure.

Worse, this stuff is in our food. One study measured the heavy metal content of conventional and organic produce and found that conventional vegetables contained higher amounts of most heavy metals as compared to their organic counterparts.[230] Organic foods have about half the cadmium of non-organic as well as less pesticide residue and higher antioxidant content.

High fat doesn't help either. It makes the effects of heavy metal toxicity worse and also inhibits removal of these metals from the body. For example, in one study volunteers drank radioactive lead either alone or with vegetable oil (it's anyone's guess why they agreed to do either). The high fat group absorbed significantly more lead than the lead alone group.[231]

Heavy Metals and Heavy Petting

We know from epidemiological studies that there are adverse reproductive associations with cadmium, lead and mercury exposure. Because of the many years of industrial use, these toxic heavy metals are ubiquitous in the environment, and now most adults have measurable amounts in our blood.[232] Thanks, Big Industry.

If you're inclined to think that surely the levels of exposure are safe, I'm sorry to point out that studies show quite the opposite. For example, metals interfere with normal puberty in females. Researchers at the National Institute of Child Health and Human Development collected blood samples from females aged six to eleven years, measuring reproductive hormones. They found that lead suppressed the production of hormones associated with puberty, especially when combined with cadmium.[233] Likewise, a study[234] of 252 healthy females who were not identified as having any particular heavy metal exposure showed that blood levels of cadmium, lead and mercury were associated with modest changes in reproductive hormones.

Yet another study[235] found that heavy metals, including mercury, cadmium, cobalt and copper adversely effected testicular cells and impaired sex hormones, including testosterone, in males.

Cadmium, mercury and lead alone have been found to adversely affect reproduction in epidemiological studies. They negatively affect the production of sex steroids.[236]Additionally, detectable levels have been found in human ovarian tissue, affecting growth of female follicles.[237]

For Robert, smoking was a clear source of cadmium exposure in his body. The resulting disruption of his hormones may have contributed to his lack of desire for sex. There are some amounts of heavy metal exposure that we have no control over, but smoking is one source that is best avoided.

Additional research shows a myriad of negative effects on sex hormones. Cadmium affects the bioavailability of both androgens and estrogens in the body.[238] Lead and mercury inhibit the binding of estradiol.[239] Epidemiological research supports that cadmium has estrogenic effects,[240] while lead is anti-estrogenic.[241] Lead is associated with delayed puberty and[242] menstruation.[243]

Arsenic poisoning and exposure to other industrial agents slows nerve conduction.[244] We know that the resultant effect on nerve impulses impairs pleasure and function. And levels of persistent organic pollutants such as polychlorinated biphenyls (PCB, commonly found in plastics) affect our hormonal health. High levels are found in many animals in the wild, suggesting a pervasive environmental exposure. One study, for example, reported that arctic foxes have high exposure to PCBs and that this can reduce their testosterone levels up to 75%.[245]

If even foxes can't outfox the impact of heavy metals on our bodies and hormones; it's clear we have to take action.

How to Deal with Metal Exposure

In a word, nature. We can look to how plants and animals adapt to metal exposure for instruction. Basically, through evolution, they've developed proteins (called metallothionein or MT and pyhtochelatin.[246]

Pharmaceutical chelating drugs failed to mimic this process and could not bring down lead levels in children with lead exposure. However, plant-based chelators, metallothioneins and phytochelatins effectively reduced lead.

MT are proteins which bind to heavy metals and are found in plants, animals and bacteria. They have the ability to protect cells from damage by free radicals and also to protect against radiation.

MTs have a big affinity for zinc in the body, but in the presence of excess cadmium or copper will bind to them instead, effectively making cells resistant to their toxicity.[247] Zinc induces MT expression, and zinc deficiency leads to a reduced ability to deal with excessive heavy metals in the body. For this reason, we should all maintain a diet with adequate zinc or supplement.

Phytochelatins also bind to metals and are produced by all higher plants and most algae. These substances protect them from the harmful effects of metal toxicity and proved in research to be *more* effective than chelating pharmaceutical drugs at removing heavy metals from the body.[248]

Our ability to deal with exposure to toxic heavy metals varies because we all have different nutritional and antioxidant status, and our bodies produce different amounts of metal-binding agents. This is why, for example, some kids develop autism following exposure to very small amounts of heavy metals[249] while most do not. Some immunologists now believe that these children's bodies are not able to launch an adequate biological response[250] to even relatively minor heavy metal exposure.

What we're really working against here is the fact that heavy metals cause oxidative stress in our bodies, on a cellular and DNA level. Because we are now exposed to more toxic heavy metals than ever, dietary antioxidants are an even more essential part of the diet, as they're proven to mitigate the negative effects of heavy metal exposure.[251]

Our particular mineral status will also determine outcomes here. The lower the dietary calcium deficit you have, the better to absorb lead and cadmium, my dear.

Increased magnesium and zinc blunted absorption of cadmium. In children, taking iron reduced lead absorption. Selenium binds to mercury in the body and helps decrease oxidative stress-related biomarkers and helps kick that mercury to the curb.[252]

And then, there are foods that seem particularly suited to carrying unwanted metals out with them. Chorella, tomatoes, moringa, cilantro, turmeric, garlic have all demonstrated the ability to show metals the door.[253] Additionally, toxic heavy metals really like sulphur, so, foods with sulphur-containing peptides such as garlic, onions and broccoli[254] are on your side.

Here is a summary of the existing research on which foods tell which metals to talk to the hand:

Cadmium
Cadmium seriously disrupts reproductive and sexual function via the endocrine system.
Cadmium Killers
• Tomatoes, berries, onions, garlic and grapes are natural antagonists to lead and cadmium thanks to their mineral content (sulphur, calcium, selenium, zinc, B vitamins, quercetin, naringenin, anthocyanin, essential elements and antioxidants). • Cadmium absorption by our intestines is reduced by increased fiber intake. Lower iron stores also contribute to higher cadmium absorption in tissues.[255] • Onion and garlic lessen cadmium-induced nephrotoxicity (toxicity of kidney tissue). Onions reduce testicular oxidative damage and improve spermatotoxicity. • Following cadmium damage, grapes improved testosterone, sperm count and motility and testicular weight.[256]

Mercury
Mercury seriously disrupts hormones and damages cells.
Mercury Killers

- Garlic protects against the cytotoxic effects of mercury on human leucocytes via its antioxidant effect,[257] vitamins C and E.[258]

- Chlorella accelerates the excretion of mercury and subsequently decreases tissue (brain and kidney) mercury levels.[259]

- Tomatoes contain substances with anti-inflammatory and anti-oxidant properties, and proteins that bind to toxic heavy metals, such as mercury, lead and cadmium, accumulation in the liver.[260]

Lead
Lead disrupts sex hormones such as testosterone and damages testicular tissue through oxidative stress. This leads to a reduction in sperm density.
Lead Killers

- Milk increases lead absorption, even skim milk, indicating that this affect is not due to the fat content.[261] Increased calcium intake though, reduces lead absorption.

- Garlic and onion considerably reduce the mean lead concentration in liver, kidneys, brain and bone tissues.[262] Garlic decreases the lead burden and restores immunological health measures in blood and tissues. Garlic removes lead where it has accumulated in tissues in people with chronic occupational lead exposure, and improved headaches, reflexes (nerve health), blood pressure and irritability.[263]

- Chlorella and ginger improve testicular damage and sperm abnormalities in mice exposed to lead.[264] So do black cumin seeds and cilantro[265] in rat testicles with lead exposure.

- Cilantro protects male testes from the effects of lead. In research, cilantro prevented testicular and sperm damage by lead. Subjects whose testes were already damaged by lead were also given cilantro, which improved damaged testicular tissue.[266]

- Black grapes protect against lead-induced oxidative stress.[267]

Arsenic
Arsenic is not just great for old lady murder mysteries, it's also a carcinogenic heavy metal that is toxic to cells, causing abnormal gene expression and damaging DNA. Arsenic kills cells by causing oxidative stress within them, slowing nerve conduction, which we know means less pleasure and sexual function.

Arsenic Killers
• The active component of turmeric, curcumin, scavenges free radicals and binds to heavy metals, protecting against heavy-metal induced liver damage.[268]
• Populations in Bangladesh exposed to high levels of arsenic due to drinking wells suffered cancers and skin diseases. Curcumin and black pepper protected this population against arsenic-induced damage to DNA.[269] Within three months, DNA levels matched the control group.[270]

The take-home message is this: we should all make a point of hitting up the local farmer market or at least the produce aisle. Fresh fruits and vegetables are our knights in shining armor with their ability to protect against so many environmental assaults. Our efforts will translate to more and better sex, increased arousal, lubrication and strong erections.

ELECTROMAGNETIC FIELDS

Now that we've started on the topic of environmental hazards, we must turn our gaze to the fields. The electromagnetic fields (EMFs). What are they? Where are they? What are they doing to us? And what can we do about it?

Electromagnetic fields in *living things* are created by moving electrical charges, or currents of electrons. Dmitry Budker, UC Berkeley professor of physics, says the human body produces tiny magnetic fields, and we can measure this electrical activity in the heart and brain with sensitive magnetometers.

Outside of our bodies, electromagnetic fields, or EMFs, come from cell phones, computers, televisions, power lines and radios, among other things. Technology we use every day, all day, and that we're around whether we're on TikTok or not.

EMFs produce electrical currents and fields. Importantly, the human body operates via electrical currents as well. For example, every time a nerve fires or the heart contracts, an electric current gets its wings.

With 5G rolling out, there has been controversy about the safety of these fields to human health. As I reviewed the medical literature of their impact on our bodies and sex lives, I saw dozens upon dozens of quality studies showing that it negatively impacts many aspects of health from our neurological, cardiovascular and immune systems, to sadly, our reproductive system. There were countless epidemiological, clinical and animal studies showing negative health effects and only a small handful failing to show such effects.

I wondered, then, why is this considered controversy at all?

Electromagnetic waves induce genetic and biological changes in the human body. This is no longer speculation, or conspiracy, as it once was, conjuring images of "crazy" people wearing tin foil hats. Interaction between the electricity of EMFs and the electricity of the human body causes known physiological disruptions. Research has shown that the level at which the average person is exposed to EMFs causes oxidative damage to DNA.[271]

That's been known within our lifetimes. As far back as 1976, Defense Intelligence Agency documents[272] reported that military personnel exposed to non-thermal microwave radiation experienced irritability, headaches, fatigue, dizziness, sleeplessness, anxiety, depression, forgetfulness and a lack of concentration.

More modern studies[273] have shown that EMFs directly increase the risk of leukemia in infants. In addition, workers[274] exposed to electromagnetic fields have an elevated risk of Alzheimer's Disease. At 2.4GHz, even Wi-Fi induces heart arrhythmia and increases blood pressure in rabbits.[275]

Radio frequency and electromagnetic radiation has demonstrated harmful effects on DNA integrity in the heart and brain.[276] Studies[277] have linked Wi-Fi exposure to neurodegenerative diseases,[278] and shown that manmade EMFs have a much stronger biological effect than natural EMFs.[279]

As of 2014, the WHO classified EMFs as being *possibly* carcinogenic to humans, though much more research has emerged since then. In a 2015 review[280] published in the *International Journal of Oncology*, scientists concluded that mobile phone radiation does cause tumors in the brain and should be regarded as a human carcinogen.

The European Environment Agency found that there was sufficient evidence that Wi-Fi exposure posed a risk of head tumors. As such they recommended we reduce exposures to EMFs, especially from mobile phones, and particularly for children and young adults, who are more susceptible to risk from head tumors.[281]

There's a possibility of accumulation of brain tissue damage from cell phone radiation.[282] This radiation causes an increase in the metabolism of glucose in the brain, which is associated with cancer.[283] Even at levels lower than the current FCC guidelines, this radiation causes biological changes in the body.

It was once thought that because levels of microwave exposure from cell phones were insufficient to cause temperature changes in the human body, that this exposure was harmless. But researchers have since found that, even one-hour, non-thermal exposure activated a stress-response in the body. This exposure changed numerous proteins in human tissues, including heat shock protein.

There's more: A 2017 study[284] concluded that long-term exposure to Wi-Fi may lead to neurogenerative disease. Any disease which damages nerves will slow and weaken signals to and from the genitals, reducing sexual pleasure and function.

In heavier patients, there is a greater vulnerability to radiation from these sources. This is likely due to hormonal differences[285] whereby a rise in estrogen leads to decreased melatonin.

Epidemiological, human and animal studies[286] on EMFs have been conducted on the male[287] and female reproductive[288] systems showing that they adversely affect the nervous and endocrine systems in regard to reproduction.

Male Reproductive System

Human and animal studies have demonstrated a significant biological impact of EMFs on the male reproductive system. Among them, EMFs lower sperm quality[289] and mobility.[290] Cell phone use induces cell death in testicular cells.[291] Sperm DNA is damaged;[292] testicular cell development is altered.[293] Exposure to 2.4GHz Wi-Fi impairs sperm function,[294] with the note that exposure in our living spaces could play a major factor in our exposure.

How do Wi-Fi and EMFs damage male sex organs? EMFs cause changes in the ultra-structure tissue of the male reproductive system, the fine structure within a cell that we can see when we use an electron microscope. EMFs interfere with intracellular calcium homeostasis, resulting in impairment of sperm function, reducing sperm motility and viability. There have been numerous studies showing that exposure to radio frequency and electromagnetic radiation significantly lowers sperm count and damages DNA.[295]

Several studies[296] have also demonstrated that exposure to EMFs induced changes in serum testosterone.

Female Reproductive System

EMFs can also disrupt the female reproductive system via the endocrine system, which alters hormonal balance, [297] affecting the uterus, ovaries and follicles.[298] This damage can reduce fertility and impair normal sexual function. Animal studies[299] have shown that neuroendocrine disorders are the main reason for fertility issues.

Prolonged exposure[300] to the electromagnetic radiation from Wi-Fi leads to oxidative stress and physiopathological changes in female reproductive structures. In animal studies,[301] exposure to EMFs from computers and TVs were enough to induce extended estrous cycles. EMFs inhibit ovulation[302] and alter growth of follicles.[303] EMFs can accelerate the process of cell death in female ovaries, too, causing the destruction of the ovarian tissue and other cells in the uterus and fallopian tubes.[304]

One study[305] found that exposure to the EMFs associated with video display terminals increased the incidence of spontaneous abortion and found a positive correlation between occupational use of monitors and fetal abnormalities. And some studies[306] have linked cell phone use to low birth weight.

EMFs can also affect implantation and fetal development. An animal study on the effects of EMFs on female reproduction demonstrated reduced fertility and embryo development because EMFs decreased the number of blastocysts and caused DNA fragmentation.[307]

Epidemiological studies[308] show that EMF-generated computer use by pregnant females increased rates of birth defects and miscarriages. The validity of these findings in humans has been debated. However, numerous studies[309] have had similar findings in animal populations.

How to Reduce Exposure to EMFs

Given that EMFs are part of our everyday lives in our homes, communities and workplaces, what possibly can we do to shield ourselves from their negative effects? There are a few simple choices[310] we can make to at least buffer or reduce our constant exposure. Here are a few:

- Use speakerphone or hands-free

- Keep calls short
- Don't wear phones
- De-activate unnecessary apps
- Use airplane mode
- Unplug cordless phone stations
- Use hard-wired ethernet internet (LAN)
- Limit use of computers, keyboards, headsets in cars and at home
- Increase water intake for detoxification
- Increase exposure to sunlight for vitamin D, which is protective

Though lacking scientific research to support its efficacy, some also recommend spending time with natural, so-called grounding electromagnetic frequencies like the woods, beach and grass.

The Earth itself emits its own EMF. And while we do know that plants, including trees, have biological electrical signaling processes, [311] scientific attempts to confirm that plants generate their own electromagnetic fields have failed. In 2009, physicists at UC Berkely tried to measure the biomagnetism of plants in the titan aurum.[312]

Every few years, this plant produces an enormous flower-like calyx with a giant phallus the size of a person plunging out of the center. It flowers for twenty-four hours only, giving it a very small window to be pollinated. In an amazing biological phenomenon, the flower heats up, reaching temperatures up to eighty-five degrees, and emits an intense odor of rotting flesh to attract flies and beetles.

Using extremely sensitive instruments, they looked for minuscule magnetic fields around the flower. Unfortunately though, they could not find a way to cancel out the local magnetic field noise, such as nearby BART trains, which interfered with the experiment. They concluded that, if the plant did produce a magnetic field, it was very very small.

Science does not yet support that plants and trees offer protection from EMFs. However, traditional Chinese medicine has viewed being in nature and taking walks in the woods as healing for thousands of years.

It's hard to believe a little time in nature isn't a safe bet.

That said, we do have some scientifically verified ways to protect ourselves from these ubiquitous EMFs. Studies have shown that increasing our antioxidants reduces the negative effects of EMF exposure.

Research shows that vitamins E and C ameliorated some of the effects[313] of cell phone radiation on cell death and oxidative stress in the uterus. Other studies[314] have confirmed this, with one[315] in particular showing that vitamin C specifically protects against oxidative damage affecting the female reproductive system.

Vitamin E is another powerful antioxidant which offers significant benefit in protecting human tissues from EMFs. Vitamin E improves the regenerative cycle, increases elasticity, converts free radicals into harmless metabolites,[316] and specifically protects male testes from certain stressors.[317] Vitamin A[318] has antioxidant properties, protecting blood platelets from damage by the EMFs of LCD monitors.

This gives us even more incentive to eat lots of fresh fruits and vegetables regularly. Melons and carrots are both excellent sources of vitamin A. Berries and other fruits, as well as potatoes, are great sources of vitamin C.

One herb that stood out for its protective effect here is fennel. Researchers believe fennel can offset the damaging effects of EMFs due to its antioxidant effects, as well as its high vitamin E and C content.[319]

Back to Robert and José, who chose to reduce their use of cell phones and increase their antioxidant intake. They ate fruit in the morning for breakfast and a vegetable-rich lunch, such as a big leafy green salad with grilled salmon.

Optimizing nutrition is great for sex in multiple ways. Not only do we nourish the qi and blood, but we also enhance the body's natural defense against environmental assault.

GREAT SEX FROM YOUR PARTNER'S EYES

A cigar is never just a cigar, and sex is never just about sex—especially within a relationship. Our attitudes and expectations, our habits and desires, are all interwoven and interdependent, and they all ladder up to what we experience sexually with a partner.

Great sex is not just about our bodies, our endurance, our sex moves, our health. It's about what's in our heads too. And right alongside all the information in this book—the diet, the acupuncture, the herbs, and the medicinals for great sex—it's essential to realize that this will only get us so far if our philosophy and attitude about sex are out of balance. If we don't understand the role of our partner's pleasure in all this, too, a better erection or more responsive clitoris is not going to make us happy in the long run. When we are selfish lovers, we are bad lovers, end-stop.

Finding that balance isn't easy for us. In our image-worshipping Western culture, the self is the center of the universe. We embrace individualism, assertiveness and endless selfies. Even today's porn is tailor-made to such impressively specific desires such that there's always a place to go for any whim without even involving a partner.

Our culture beats a steady of drum of messages to focus on how to meet our needs, our expectations and our satisfaction in every way. This perspective may be great for a confidence boost, but it's a disaster in the bedroom, where eagerness to please is the only argument that wins the day.

In other words, it's not enough to care for our own bodies. We may eat as healthy as possible and log hours of exercise, mastering the physiology of a good lay. But if we don't think beyond ourselves, we won't have great sex, and neither will our partner.

Mark My Words

Take Mark. Mark wanted more than anything to find a partner who would love him unconditionally. Yet, in examining his practices in his relationships, it was clear why that wasn't happening. He was so focused on his own needs that every person he fell for ended up leaving him.

For instance, he preferred to split the bill on dates right down the middle. When he did pay, he expected her to really take notice, often forgetting that she paid at times too. Rather than see the acts of intimacy and connection from his partner, he had a narrative in his mind that portrayed him as extremely generous and benevolent and others as suspicious, taking advantage of his generosity. He sometimes reminded women he dated as he plopped down that card for the bill that he wasn't a sugar daddy (oof).

Naturally, he bolstered this stance with personal philosophies about how people should act. Mark thought that people should be self-sufficient (like him!) and not impose on others. When his partner asked him to help her move, he thought she was really asking a lot. He lectured her to be considerate of other people's time by leaving him out of it and hiring a moving company. When he did end up helping, just as with paying for dinner, he made another big show of his generosity, never missing an opportunity to remind her of his act of kindness.

So it should surprise exactly no one that in bed, there was only one position that Mark liked—doggie style—and so that was the position they would always have sex in. He said that all of the other ones were uncomfortable, even though he was a healthy young man with no medical issues. He also liked it when his partner gave him oral, but he wasn't really into reciprocating, as he said he was sensitive to smells and prone to nausea. It never occurred to him that this was a gross imbalance of pleasure, nor did he ever wonder if his partner's actual needs were met.

Some of this stuff, it must be said, is about our antiquated notions of gender. Typically, men are conditioned to see the world as a treasure trove of pleasure aimed directly at them via sexualized images of women of all types at every turn. Women are often taught to cater to male pleasure, utterly disregarding their own.

Times are changing though. And it would be unfair to paint men as the only ones who are self-centered. Plenty of women are selfish in bed and selfish in relationships. Likewise, lots of men are exceedingly generous lovers. Regardless of gender or identity, we, as human beings, innately think about our own well-being and must teach ourselves the virtue of giving.

Mark's attitude made him a bit of a dinosaur in his dating life in an era where men are now far more eager to please women and discover the pathways to their pleasure. Given that the entirety of his thoughtfulness around sex was the expectation that his partners completely accommodate him at the expense of their own pleasure, they eventually tired of this and moved on to someone who was kinder to their needs, or someone who, unlike Mark, was even remotely curious about what those needs even looked like.

Incredibly, Mark had another invented belief system to explain the relationship's demise: He chose to believe conveniently that partners kept leaving him because his penis wasn't large enough. Second thought: Maybe he just wasn't rich enough for these gold diggers.

But eventually, he tired of the cycle too. Frustration, unending horniness and heartbreak will do that to you. So after many failed partnerships, he began to do a self-inventory. He was reminded of something that many friends and lovers had told him, that he was selfish, and for once, chose to really explore that notion.

In his suffering, he developed humility. He sought ways to be a better person, including learning how to pleasure his partner sexually. He decided that with his next partner, he would make sure that their pleasure came first. And when he finally began to think about his partner's needs, both in the relationship and sexually, he found a relationship that lasted.

As we see in this example, selfishness is rarely isolated to just a smash-and-dash in the bedroom. It is usually apparent both in sex and in the day-to-day of the relationship. Mark wanted his needs to be met but didn't consider his partner's needs.

Remember, both yin *and* yang are part of great sex. Without yin, yang cannot exist, as they are born of each other. When we nourish our counterpart, our minds can merge, leading to sex that is more engaged. And by freeing up the mind from self-oriented thoughts we can more fully experience the sensations of sex.

Unexpected Education

In working with my patients for acupuncture and dietary health, I have learned a tremendous amount of information about people's relationships. When I treat people for sexual health, they usually start by telling me about problems with their partner. Though the details are always different, they are strikingly similar, essentially all complaining of the *same* problem.

That problem is this: They don't feel cared for by their partner.

All human beings long to be nurtured. It is established in childhood by a loving caregiver. While the desire for nurturing is the same, what that looks like differs among individuals. Psychology has come at this in numerous ways, explaining it as compatibility, love languages, communication skills and more.

But the point is this: We all have to find out what makes our partner feel nurtured, and then go do it. For some people, that's making them a pot roast; for others, it's copious amounts of oral.

Libido, Labado

Physiological differences in males and females, not to mention enormous, pervasive cultural messages exaggerating those differences beyond all reality, have left us with the general belief that men, de facto, have higher libidos than women.

You've likely heard this all your life: Men are total horndogs and women would just as soon read an IKEA manual. Jokes about women not putting out once the wedding is complete abound. The idea here is that women have sex at first to lock a guy down, and then reveal her true, maternal, frigid self, who never actually liked sex in the first place.

The truth is far more complex than our biased brains can grasp, and much new research suggests that things are not quite so predictable. In fact, they may be entirely flipped. Female libidos are not only present and active but may far outrun those of males in some ways. Modern research[320] says female lust has been underestimated (and repressed) for 1,500 years. In fact, when women's *physiological* response was measured, it revealed they were far more aroused than they reported, and by a wider variety of sexual stimuli, including sex with strangers, for instance.

Much of the long-assumed lower libido of women may really be about cultural repression and lack of female orgasm in many modern relationships. Imagine never getting off in a relationship with someone who doesn't know how to do it, or who doesn't care, or who doesn't consider your orgasm important, then being told the real problem is you're just not lusty enough. Over time, you'd be conditioned not to expect real pleasure and would lose interest. That tends to be a common experience of many women in heterosexual relationships.

But all that taken together still leaves us with this result: I see, as many sexual health experts do, far more patients where men present with a higher sex drive and women seem prone to a lower one, and this difference can wreak havoc on relationships.

Complaint Box

As a result of this disparity, countless men complain to me that their partner is not very interested in sex. Regardless of why that's happening, these men often feel sad and lonely without being able to share that intimacy.

In any pairing where desire and libido do not match, there will be great frustration, sadness and loneliness. This has given me a particularly deep compassion for men in treating them for sexual health. As a result, part of my work is helping them explore the root of their partner's lack of interest and discovering the possibility of great sex for both of them. (Hint: It's not the same position all the time where the woman never gets off).

Again, males aren't the only ones who are horny. Women need sex too. So, regardless of orientation or identity, many people are dissatisfied in their relationships simply because their partners aren't having enough sex with them. What enough means though, is highly individual. But for most people, feeling nurtured fundamentally includes being cared for sexually, and nothing is going to change that.

Mismatched Libido

Taken together, we can draw one true conclusion: Mismatched libido is a really tough problem for any relationship because one person feels nagged and the other feels neglected.

For those with a high libido, regular sex is an essential part of their sense of well-being in a relationship. It is likely to be tied to self-esteem and feelings of connection with a partner. I have seen many divorces where one partner's sole complaint was lack of sex, with the person feeling chronically rejected and alone.

For the partner whose libido is lower, they get tired of constantly being a disappointment. They feel they shouldn't have to apologize for a physical difference. And this constant pressure to perform can, over time, develop into a negative association with sex in general.

Often, this devolves into a disagreement about how much sex is normal in a relationship. If it's any consolation, experts have the same argument. What constitutes a "normal" amount of sex is a hotly contested point of debate even within psychology.

The old adage that we should all do it twice a week is a bit misleading—it's drawn from research showing that happy couples have sex about twice a week, so it became the advice typically given to couples who don't have sex at all. The twice a week goal is recommended as a starting point to ensure a frequent physical connection and intimacy. A sexual midpoint if you will.

Individual frequency preference, though, is another matter. One woman's constant is another man's never.

For instance, one female patient of mine said that she would be happy if her wife wanted to have sex a couple times a month. Another guy complained that his wife only had sex with him every Friday.

One guy was resentful that he and his partner didn't do it every day. His partner did the best she could to keep up, averaging five times per week (!) even after twenty years of marriage. She tried so hard to make him happy, and still he wasn't satisfied. He ended up leaving her for a younger woman (to whom we'd love to send our condolences).

The likelihood that your partner's libido matches exactly to yours is slim. But that doesn't mean this thing is doomed. Kindness, curiosity, patience, understanding and of course, TALKING ABOUT IT by both people can help suss out what makes for a happy, horny compromise needed to maintain harmony despite these differences.

What Your Partner Really Wants

What *does* your partner want? Well, sex. Maybe that pot roast. Oral. Some cuddling. Maybe a bit of kink. There's only one way to find out: ask. Even if you think you know, ask anyway. Pay close attention to the details too. No one needs to come home wanting a quickie only to find a whole sex dungeon obstacle course set up.

That is, what we *think* a partner wants may be quite different from what they really want. Just as what looks good and feels good varies.

Open Your Mind and Your Ham Wallet

This reminds me of something. I was in an airport one day when I saw a poster for gynecological cosmetic surgery, which, as it tends to do, invoked my ire.

Women have enough insecurities to worry about after a lifetime of messaging to shave our vag, legs and pits, to hoist it up with wires, to plumpen our boobs, to haul it through time and space on stilts, to lengthen our legs and prop up our asses. It's exhausting. Now we need vaginal cosmetic surgery too?

Women live with a steady chorus in our heads telling us we aren't going to be attractive to a partner because we don't have a big enough butt or our boobs are too small or our teeth are crooked or we've got a gut.

So when I saw that ad I thought, *Do women really think that surgically mutilating their genitals will make them more fuckable?* The answer, sadly, is that yes, some do believe this.

Now, I'm not here to tell women they can't improve themselves as they please, and some alterations can be part of a healthy self-image. But I wanted to take what I saw on the plastic surgeon's website—a highlight reel of before-and-afters of vulvas—to heart and to the streets. I wanted to find out if people would validate their expensive, costly and potentially response-damaging efforts as needed.

Some of the women were concerned that the labia minora, or the smaller lips, extended outside of the labia majora, or larger lips, and they had these corrected. I know from my practice that the appearance of a partner's labia to the quality of sex or arousal is insignificant for most people, yet here were all these women willing to surgically alter their genitals because they thought it was important. (Ahem, the reason is usually the widespread, pervasive availability of porn.)

What these women may not have realized is that, even if *they* don't like the looks of their genitals, they may look quite attractive to their partners. From talking with so many men and women about these issues, I have realized that insecurities about the minor aesthetics of one's genitals are usually unfounded.

Vulvas are like faces in that each is unique. My boyfriend said that he would definitely be able to identify mine in a police lineup. He also said that seeing a woman naked for the first time is exciting, not an opportunity to practice a *Where's Waldo* of flaws.

You don't know from looking at a clothed woman how her breasts and nipples will look, or her labia. There's not one standardized look that is more attractive. In fact, the consensus is that they *all* are attractive, and it's both exciting and arousing to see the uniqueness of a person's genitals.

As I perused the before pics of the women's genitals, I saw that each one looked perfectly normal and each unique. There were bald vulvas and super hairy vulvas. The labia were all unique sizes and proportions. One reminded me of an Arby's roast beef sandwich. They each looked right just the way they were, and I certainly couldn't see why these women felt so bad that they would want to go through surgery.

So, I conducted an informal poll. Less than scientifically, I asked some heterosexual male friends of mine, my boyfriend and two lesbians to look at the pics. Their responses were quite interesting. First of all, none thought the after pics looked *any* more attractive than the before pics. Not one bit.

Secondly, *all* of the males said that the sight of all of these female genitals was quite arousing, just as they were. This was not porn, per se. No lacy thongs or powdery lighting and on a backdrop of an exam table with florescent lighting and paper hospital gowns.

The sandwich-like vulva in the before photos had lots of ridges and folds on the labia majora, with the labia minora curling far outside of the labia majora. One friend looked at it and said, "Oh, this is lovely!" He was *especially* aroused by this less-common female genitalia. Had the woman in this photo known how much her vulva could arouse a person, perhaps she would have thought twice about surgically altering it. I would also be concerned about scar tissue forming from the surgery and if this would cause pain or reduced blood flow and sensitivity later on, so I'm not strictly discussing looks here.

Neither lesbian thought the pics, with their clinical lighting and framing, were at all arousing, but they thought they looked perfectly normal. Of course, this was not scientific data but merely anecdotal.

But this anecdata is intended to say this: What we *think* a partner wants is very different from what they actually want. What looks good is entirely different than what feels good too. And the lion's share of our insecurities about these live only in our heads.

Sausage Party

The same could be said for the vast, pervasive male fear about penis size. Men, too, have been fed a pornlike stream of giant penises their whole lives and increasingly express deep-seated fears that they are simply not adequate. All the dick jokes don't help, and society tends to use this against men in some pretty sick burns about smaller penis size explaining nearly every unattractive male behavior on earth.

Men overwhelmingly exaggerate their penis size, but that goes both ways. They either think it's bigger than it is (or rather, they lie) or they fear it's too small when in fact it's average. In other words, all this stuff has messed with their heads too, and they have no idea what women really like either.

I can tell you what they like: To feel pleasure, and to get off. Research shows that women are far less concerned with size when it comes to how they rank satisfaction with men than performance. In other words, if women report unhappiness in a relationship, it's rarely because he's not big enough; it's because she doesn't orgasm.

The only research that suggests bigger is better is for one-night stands. One study found that women did prefer a larger penis if they never intended to see it again. Research shows that many hetero women like an average-sized penis, particularly for long-term commitment. It's not too big as to be painful, nor is it too small to be pleasurable. There's even a term for it in pop culture: Boyfriend Dick. But a guy being great in bed *truly* has nothing to do with his size. He simply knows how to pleasure his partner.

It's the Chemistry, Stupid

We all have preferences, sure, but most of us can find someone attractive who is well outside of them. The reason is that it's one thing to judge a person by the picture only (looking at you, Tinder) but quite another to connect with someone.

We worry that we aren't good-looking enough, smart enough, hung enough, stacked enough or successful enough. But we forget that most of us just want to find someone we have chemistry with.

Yes, size matters, but you don't need an anaconda.

The problem is that we remember that *one* person who made us feel insecure and then generalize this to everyone. I remember this guy I dated who would drool over women with big asses. I have a small, European-bred ass that's kind of square, if I'm being honest. Ever since then I felt insecure about it. My friend though, has a huge, sexy ass, but she feels bad because her boobs are small.

One guy told me he felt insecure because he is really short and lots of women on Tinder said they wouldn't go out with a short guy. Another guy was considering surgical implants to make his penis longer.

Our insecurities are very powerful motivators, driving us to do all sorts of crazy things like surgery. The truth is that there are loads of us who aren't that superficial, looking more at what kind of connection we have with a person. Many potential mates care more about how kind a person is and how they will be treated. A male friend of mine openly says, "I may have a small dick, but I'm really good at eating pussy." Hey, having that skill-set alone is good enough for me, and I would say good enough for most women.

Unfortunately, we spend a lot of time wondering if we are good enough. But insecurities can make you a kinder, more humble person. When we have this humility we can be more compassionate with our partner.

As a society we really need this kind of seismic shift. Each of us has unique gifts meant to help others and bring joy to their lives. Ironically, it is in focusing on others that we bring joy to our own lives. This fosters more loving relationships and better sex.

Social media has its fingerprints all over this crime scene. It has completely changed the world of love and sex. What would once have been considered self-obsessed is the new norm, as everyone snaps constant pics of themselves at every angle imaginable and at every time and place, translating what was once personhood into a full-fledged brand.

Image seems more important than substance as we try to present a picture to others that our lives are exciting and fulfilling even if they are far from it. And as we spend more time looking at a screen and less having actual conversations, we've lost our game. Young men and women are finding it harder to connect in this new age of screen interactions. Some dating apps have made the process easier though, but not without that initial hurdle of lookist obsession that means for every gained opportunity based on delighting in a head shot, there's more lost ones due to shallow swiping.

Respect and Kindness

So far, we've discussed the way mismatched libido gets in the way of even healthy, enthusiastic partners. But often libido is not the obvious culprit we think it is. What I've come across often in my work with clients is that we, as human beings, sometimes lack basic kindness in our relationships, and nothing will kill a relationship faster than not being nice to one another.

Partners who don't feel well cared for are far less likely to desire intimate acts with someone who has caused them pain. That seems so obvious as to not need be stated, but here we are.

I don't think anyone starts out intending to steamroll their partner's feelings and concerns, but sure enough, over time, the little acts of kindness, love and nurturing sometimes erode or vanish either because of familiarity, bickering, real betrayals or just the cumulative result of a backlog of unresolved issues and bad experiences.

Couples who truly have respect, kindness and love for each other also have better sex. They nurture each other inside and outside of the bedroom, and that connection and effort is rewarded at every level.

You simply can't expect great, connective, satisfying sex without caring about how someone feels in every aspect of their lives. For that, we must manage our own expectations and understand the expectations of our partner. Using the strategies in this book can significantly improve sex, but only if both partners are willing to try.

That respect and nourishment for body and mind, being inseparable, are central tenets of traditional Chinese medicine.

They are also tenets of its practitioners.

Every time I treat a patient, I silently recite this simple prayer: "Dear God, please heal this beautiful child." It's a reminder that the person who lies on the table before me is my only focus in this moment, deserving my undivided attention, compassion and love, and that requires listening to them, taking in the story of their current existence to understand why they came to see me.

While the efficacy of praying is well established in research, that's not the point of it. The point is that every person needs kindness, love and nurturing, including your partner.

Humility

In traditional Chinese medicine, the mind is considered inseparable from physical health. Our emotions of anger, fear, sadness, joy and worry can both cause disease and be the product of it.

In TCM, the state of having unbalanced emotions is believed to be both a symptom of and a cause of disease. For example, let's take the emotion of anger. Anger provokes illnesses of the liver. In turn, liver problems, cause excessive anger. You can visualize this in someone with liver yang rising, causing high blood pressure. This disruption may have been caused by anger or be causing anger in the patient.

This association has also been established in conventional medical research. Studies have found that anger and hostility are associated with coronary heart disease.[321] Fear is the emotion associated with the kidneys, worry with the spleen, joy with the heart, and grief with the lungs. By caring for our bodies physically, we also care for ourselves emotionally, which supports healthy relationships.

It's ok to be human, and we all make mistakes. We might snap at our partner when they try to help us. Sometimes we act selfishly or we don't do our share because we feel tired. Maybe we get wrapped up in the stress of life and forget to be loving and affectionate. But most relationship issues can be worked through if we communicate with our partner in a kind way.

To do that, we need humility in spades.

Humility would stop us before we overestimate our contributions to a relationship and under-appreciate our partner's. It helps us avoid magnifying our hurt and minimizing our partner's.

Without humility, we arrogantly expect our partners not to have major flaws, even though we ourselves are human and have major flaws. And to top all that off, we don't seem to see our own flaws as clearly as we see those of our partner.

Humility teaches us to temper our emotions. When life is stressful, each of us has certain go-to emotions drawn from our earliest experiences, past relationships, and lifelong accumulated habits for how we process and handle our feelings. For some of us, anger and irritability is the first emotion we feel under stress. Some of us sink into depression, others anxiety.

But harnessing humility, and gratitude, the latter of which we must learn to express out loud with actual words, is the buffer against those self-centered ways of being.

What does this look like?

To start, we would deliver criticism with love behind our words, instead of anger and judgment. Instead of "I think you're an asshole for doing X, Y and Z," we don't see our partners as assholes at all but human beings who make mistakes.

To follow, we'd also receive criticism better and with more kindness, even if it wasn't expressed perfectly, as an opportunity to hear how our partner is suffering and to relieve that suffering. If they say that they don't feel appreciated, that you hurt their feelings, or that they would like you to touch them differently in bed, try to listen with an open mind and don't get defensive. Be kind, even though criticism can sting.

My aunt recently told me that "hurt people hurt people." In other words, when we feel hurt, we hurt others. Recognizing this in ourselves and in others can help us to be kinder. Humility, which renders us as students still learning and growing, capable of mistakes but worthy of love, is the only way through this problem.

Kindness extends to the bedroom as well. When we regard our partner as an equal, we realize that we must focus on their sexual pleasure as much as our own, and kindness dictates we do so with open minds, curiosity and decency. When both yin and yang are happy, sex is harmoniously delightful.

APHRODISIACS: FLUFFERS OF THE GODS

We've talked about the literal sex foods that will improve blood flow and vascular function, sometimes within mere hours. Now let's consider the humble complementary foods and spices that lead to spicier sex. Aphrodisiacs.

Aphrodisiacs are nature's culinary firecrackers, the herbs, spices, foods and medicinals that put the pep back in your sexual step, the O back in your libido. Aphrodisiacs get a lot of play in the culture at large, from listicles detailing oysters and essential oils, to more figurative notions that incite lust. For some people, a sense of humor is the biggest aphrodisiac in town, for others (ahem, men), rejection. An old saying suggests a woman's aphrodisiac is in her ears (get it? being listened to!); another famous joke indicates that anyone who thinks the way to a man's heart is through his stomach must've flunked geography.

Those are all illuminating thoughts, but I'm talking about the kind of aphrodisiacs you actually eat.

Broadly defined as substances that strengthen sexual desire, pleasure or function, aphrodisiacs are often dismissed as lacking any scientific evidence whatsoever. As such, we see images in pop culture of sex potions and snake-oil gimmicks, where some unwitting chap is dosed unawares (a dubious form of seduction) with a swig of Horny Goat Weed that instantly transforms him into an insatiable, lust-crazed animal.

In fact, many aphrodisiacs have been studied scientifically. And taken together, there's enough evidence to explain why certain foods have been relied upon throughout to ages to gently stir the loins toward heightened pleasure. They're not, I repeat, not, an instant-fix, some zero-to-sixty gas pedal on the lust meter.

You can't blame us for wanting them to be, though, and for our resulting skepticism about their efficacy. After all, the backstory on the stuff doesn't help their scientific cred.

The word aphrodisiac itself comes from mythology, specifically a strangely erotic story of Aphrodite, goddess of love, beauty and sex, that involves tossing around genitals and frothing sea water.

It starts when Titan Cronus butchers his father, Uranus, ruler of the universe, and rudely chucks his genitals into the waters of Paphos on the island of Cypress. Then, out of the foam, arises the sensual Aphrodite. As you'd expect from anyone who was quite literally formed from a god's penis and foam, Aphrodite is a pretty horny gal. She took many lovers in her time and didn't shy away from dalliances with men and gods alike.

Making credibility matters more interesting, over the years, what passes for an aphrodisiac gets pretty unusual, including animal penis and testicles, rhinoceros horn, silkworm extract and even human placenta.

Probably the most famous aphrodisiac is Spanish fly, which is in fact a real substance made from blister beetles. History is rich with accounts of Spanish fly being used as an aphrodisiac. Roman emperor Augustus Caesar's wife was said to have used it to encourage sexual indiscretion among her guests, information which she would later use to blackmail them. Spanish fly was widely used among French royalty in the 1600s. The French sorceress, La Voisin used it to make love potions and mixed it with bat and mole blood.

In the 1700s, French writer, Marquis de Sade, used and bred the Spanish fly for use in his brothel. That didn't work out so hot: He was sentenced to death for nearly killing two prostitutes with anise-flavored Spanish fly tablets in preparation for an orgy.

Madame du Barry, King Louis XV's mistress, gave Spanish fly to young girls to prepare them for sex with the aging king (*shudder*).[322] Of course, the pursuit of great sex came with some risks. In fact, Spanish fly has had countless fatalities over the ages.

There are, however, plenty of aphrodisiacs that have some science to back their efficacy, and many of them are culinary herbs and spices which can easily be incorporated into the diet.

For example, there's delightful saffron. Its fragrant rush clearly packs a punch, as it's used frequently to flavor Middle Eastern, Indian and Grecian dishes, such as rice, and for thousands of years in Eastern medicine to spice teas and foods. You could find it in perfumes and ointments and as a brilliant yellow dye. It's a mood booster, too, often sprinkled on a bed or in tea for those who were feeling downhearted.

Whatever it did, it did it frighteningly well because travelers to Persia were once warned against eating saffron-laced dishes, such as rice, believing they could be drugged with this potent aphrodisiac.

In Ancient Egypt, Cleopatra used half a cup of saffron (which, frankly, is a lot) in her warm baths and before sex to enhance pleasure. Alexander the Great also bathed in saffron water to relieve the aches and pains of battle. These tales are dusted like saffron throughout mythology, like the one where the nymph turned her suitor into the Crocus plant with only the huge stamen to remind us that he was once a man (*that*'ll show him). Elsewhere, everyone from goddesses to monkeys picked saffron, and mythical sailors went on dangerous voyages to seek riches bestowed only by this precious herb.

Saffron was even woven into ancient royal Persian rugs. It was offered to deities. When the Black Death spread throughout Europe in the 1300s, saffron was in the highest demand for its medicinal properties. Pirates were known to favor saffron loads over gold. And the fourteen-week Saffron War began over the theft of 800 pounds of saffron from Swiss merchants by noblemen.

It turns out that all this hype is warranted. In research, saffron improved multiple measures of sexual function, desire and pleasure in both males and females.

Herbs, Foods, and Spices, and Everything Nices

Below is a glossary of the substances actually studied, while including a few of the most famous aphrodisiacs in history, regardless of their scientific backing, because you can't talk about aphrodisiacs without them. We can file away the rest for trivia night with our coworkers.

As always, a word of caution: When messing around with sexual potency, be careful what you wish for because you just might get it. Aphrodisiacs, like seances, are not to be fooled with by the unserious. You don't want to open a demon portal in your home and certainly not in your bathroom. You should have the same equal fear of an unending boner with Viagra that you would for the agonizing effects of too much Spanish fly (in the case of the latter, fear of dying).

Since aphrodisiacs haven't been *widely* researched for safety and efficacy, and some of them lack *human* studies, we should apply the same common sense we do with any medicinal we're hoping will give us animal endurance.

There are no standardized dosages when it comes to this stuff. Many of us mistakenly think that if a little is good, then a lot is better, and when it comes to nature's little fluffers, even simple culinary herbs and spices, that is a recipe for disaster.

For the stronger stuff, consult a knowledgeable herbalist who can tailor dosages to you. That way, including them in your diet for great sex will be less cartoon and more erotica.

Here's is a sample traditional aphrodisiac recipe from *The Kamasutra:*

> *"Smash together equal parts of cinnamon and green nutmeg. Add double the quantity of fresh ginger root. Add nine beans of black pepper, two to three cloves, and a teaspoon of saffron. Allow the mixture to infuse for three days in 250g of alcohol at 60 degrees. When this process is complete, add 25mg of ginseng root. Consume three teaspoons of this aphrodisiac 30 minutes before every meal."*[323]

Culinary Aphrodisiacs

African ginger *Siphonochilus aethiopicus.*
    This fragrant culinary root is used to flavor African dishes. It can increase sperm count,[324] but also treats depression and increases libido,[325] which is why it's often called Women's Viagra. Bonus: It also decreases cell damage,[326] but eat it for the libido part.

Almonds *Prunus dulcis.*
    Originating in Asia, almonds spread in popularity to Israel, Morocco, Spain and Greece. They've since found worldwide stardom, so pure in nutritional content they're even mentioned in the Christian

Bible. Newlyweds in ancient Rome were given almonds to promote fertility, and the ultimate sex guide, *The Kamasutra*, gives almonds an aphrodisiac shout-out.

Medicine has thrown them a bone too: Almonds have shown the ability to reverse some effects of diabetes,[327] which causes significant drops in nitric oxide, testosterone and certain hormones. They also increase sperm count and motility.[328]

Black pepper *Piper Nigrum.*

Black pepper is an aphrodisiac, and it's also—wait for it—a fruit. It originates from an evergreen vine native to the Malabar Coast in India, and we've been consuming and using this berry in dried form in a wide range of activities since at least 2000 BCE.

It was good enough for the pharaohs: Ramses the Great's (1303-1213 BC) mummified remains were found with peppercorns in his nose. Unless there's a sex thing I'm unaware of, that's not exactly our purpose here. Our purpose is this: In research, black pepper significantly increased sexual desire and performance.[329]

Chile peppers *Capsicum annuum.*

Chile peppers are a kink fan's dream. They're one of the only foods to physiologically produce pain but also bring us pleasure to eat. That gets our mouths watering, though for the plant, it protects them from predators, fungus and other microbes.

The Incas and Mayans used them as currency, and they go way back: Chile pepper seeds from as much as 6,000 years ago have been found in Mexico and Peru. Aztecs and Mayans used chiles culinarily, as medicine and to fumigate homes. Christopher Columbus brought the first chile peppers to the rest of the world, and a quarter of the world's population now eats them daily.

There are wild claims about their sexual potency. *The Kamasutra,* for instance, claims that if a male penetrates a female after having rubbed a mixture of long peppers and black pepper mixed in honey on his penis, she will be subject to his will. (His will must have been for her to run away screaming). But honestly this sounds a lot like today's warming lubricant.

According to research, there may be a nonsexual explanation for why we enjoy this pain-producing plant so much. Capsaicin, which ironically, is used to relieve pain, and which forms the spicy substance, activates our dopamine reward pathway through the brain's central opioid system.[330] That combination of ouch, then ahhh, explains the pepper's unique pain-pleasure dynamic. Chiles are also vitamin-packed hotshots, including vitamins A, C, K, B6, as well as potassium, iron, magnesium, copper, manganese, thiamin, riboflavin, niacin, folate and phosphorus. (This won't be on the test.)

Capsaicin has also shown to significantly enhance testicular cell growth and increase testosterone.[331] Other studies showed that it promotes vascular and metabolic health,[332] which is precisely the sexual function result we're putting ourselves through all this for.

But this really doesn't have to hurt: My preferred way to eat chile peppers is in a homemade salsa and guacamole, which also has fresh lime, garlic and onions, all of which, no surprise, confer even more aphrodisiac benefits. (Keep the kink in the bedroom.)

Chinese leeks *Allium tuberosum.*

Chinese leeks proved in at least one study to contain sex-enhancing properties, and they also stimulated sexual arousal. Pretty good for a humble leek. Other research found that they increase concentrations of testosterone.[333] Their seeds significantly improve our seed, with additional research finding that they increase sperm viability and sperm count. So leek alive, and get some leeks in your diet.

Chocolate *Theobroma cacao.*

Chocolate is a no-brainer for sex—you can conjure its velvety richness on command at the mere mention of the word, as if your mouth is being *seduced on the inside*—but it always feels good to be reminded to eat it. It also has a more lurid history than you might realize. Native to Latin America, Mayans once traded cacao beans for sex. Technically that's because they used the beans as a form of currency, but I think we've all been horny enough to get there ourselves.

It's also, unsurprisingly, a gift from god. Well, a gift from the ancient god Quetzalcoatl, the god of wisdom. Its use dates back thousands of years. Aztecs, always the clever builders, combined chocolate with vanilla to excite the passions even more. Montezuma—remember him from Social Studies? Big Aztec ruler, happened to really, really like human sacrifice? Montezuma was said to consume upwards of fifty cups of chocolate a *day* to satisfy all of his wives, and I think we can easily imagine what happened when he couldn't. Luckily, we try to keep our wives to the minimum these days, so no need to get carried away on the chocolate.

Weirdly, several studies *failed* to demonstrate that chocolate was an effective aphrodisiac. A 2006 study, for example, came back with zero evidence of sex-enhancing excellence on the chocolate front.[334]

Regardless of that oddity, chocolate does have a secret weapon in phenylethylamine, a substance which can excite us and increase our sense of well-being. Since being excited and feeling good are also words we would use to describe sex (at least, the good kind), it's easy to see how chocolate pulls off the amazing feat of indirectly relaxing our inhibitions toward sex. That's right: Chocolate actually loosens us up for doing it. And to think, you thought you needed booze for that.

Cloves *Syzygium aromatium.*

Goth teens love smoking them in cigarette form, and wars were once fought over them. If you ever take in this intoxicatingly fragrant spice you'll know why.

Our ancestors used cloves for a wide variety of purposes. Chinese emperors in the Han Dynasty, for instance, elevated hygiene etiquette by making anyone who addressed them to first chew cloves to freshen their breath.

They don't just freshen breath, though, they spark violence. The Spice Wars, or the Dutch-Portugese War, happened because the

Maluku Islands of Indonesia, a.k.a., The Spice Islands, were the only place on Earth to grow cloves, nutmeg and mace. When the rest of the world got a taste of cloves, people were crazy to get their hands on the rights to these spices. But cloves can also stir up our sexual passions.

Here, research lends the assist: One study found a significant increase in sexual desire and performance in as little as one hour after eating them.[335] Other research found they increase testosterone.[336]

To get some of that clove action, consider getting cozy with a luxuriantly rich baklava—flakey pastry filled with clove, cinnamon, cardamom and walnuts, and then topped with rose water honey.

Dates *Phoenix dactylifera.*

Need a date? Eat a date. Dates do have a sexy story. They're likely from a place called the Fertile Crescent (near Mesopotamia), for date's sake. They're experienced too: Dates are the oldest cultivated fruit in the world. There is evidence they were used back as early as 6000 BC by early Hebrews, who turned them into bread, wine and vinegar.

They're packed with nutritional accolades, from vitamins, minerals and antioxidants, and the Ajwa date has been found to reduce testicular damage from toxins in food, enhancing sperm production and testicular structure along the way.[337] Date fruit is particularly useful and can mature the sperm and improve testosterone[338] and other hormones.

Dates protect reproductive structures from oxidative stress in adults, and their mineral content improves hormone balance and protects women's eggs.[339] Even the pollen of the date palm gets in on the action improving sperm count, motility, morphology and DNA quality.

And, if you're interested in this sort of thing, let's just get this out there: They also increase testicular weight. That's right: Want big balls? Eat dates.

Dill *Anethum graveolens.*

Dill is great for your pickle. The Bible said so. Not exactly, but they did mention it. It was used in Egypt 5,000 years ago. Babylonians were growing it in their gardens in 3000 BC. Greeks, pioneers of various oils for consumption and pleasure, flavored wines with dill. Romans thought it would make their gladiators more courageous (then again, they also drank bone ash tonics).

Children were given dill seeds to calm hunger pains, and taxes on dill even paid for repairs on the London Bridge in the 1300s. Dill was believed to have magical protective properties against witchcraft and curses, and it was also added to love potions and aphrodisiacs.[340] Modern research has not just shown that dill is safe for consumption, it also happens to increase sexual desire in males.[341]

Think about all that next time you see dill winking at you from a menu in the many culinary dishes it appears in around the world, and maybe start adding it to your own homemade salad dressings. You know—*wink*—for flavor.

Fennel *Foeniculum vulgare.*

Fennel, native to Europe and the Mediterranean, is another multi-faceted sex food. It was hung over doors in the Middle Ages to ward off spirts. Used by Ancient Egyptians as food and medicine and in China for snake bites.

Thanks to vitamin C and phytoestrogens, it benefits female health[342] so reliably that when made into a vaginal cream, it increases arousal, wetness, orgasm and satisfaction and decreases pain.[343] It soothes a host of female reproductive ailments including intensely bad periods, PMS, premature loss of a period, menopause, PCOS and even quells menopause symptoms such as hot flashes, vaginal dryness and itching. That, in turn, improves sexual satisfaction, as well as the only thing better than sexual satisfaction, a good night's sleep.[344] In another study,[345] fennel improved measures of overall reproductive health.

Fennel oil has anti-inflammatory, antimicrobial, antioxidant and antispasmodic properties. It also aids in our body's hormone synthesis. And important for us, the seeds are high in naturally occurring nitrates, and baby, we know what those do: blood flow to the genitals. It doesn't ignore male function either: For that, fennel ups total protein concentration in the seminal vesicles and prostate.

Speaking of upped seminal vesicles, can I offer you some Italian sausage? No really. Fennel is a principal seasoning in Italian sausage. I add half a cup of fennel seeds (this is for a *large* pot) and half a teaspoon nutmeg to my Sunday sauce, along with a handful of fresh parsley and some chiles, which imparts that same sausage flavor. If that's not your jam, put a little fennel bulb in your minestrone soup.[346]

Fenugreek *Trigonellae semen.*

To start, *semen* is already in the Latin form of this word.

Similarly, the fenugreek herb is warm and bitter. In your body, it enters the liver and kidney channels. There, it warms the kidney yang, expels cold and relieves pain for impotence, low libido and pain in the testicles.

The Kamasutra makes a particular mention of it as an early prescription for breast enlargement. That's not surprising, as in research it's shown to increase milk flow for nursing breasts in as little as twenty-four hours, as well as improve libido and other measures of sexual function.

Figs *Ficus carica.*

Figs have been on the aphrodisiac list since day one. Stone tablets record the culinary use of figs by Sumerians in 2500 BC. Major religions can't get enough of figs either. They're signs of fertility in Buddhism, Christianity and Islam, and Greeks also associated them with sexuality.

What's more, some historians believe that the forbidden fruit in the Garden of Eden was actually the fig, not the apple that tempted Eve. (Though interestingly in *Genesis*, Adam and Eve famously used fig leaves to cover up their nakedness out of shame. Apples wouldn't have quite gotten the job done).

In ancient Rome, figs were regarded as a symbol of the female genitalia and were gifted as both a blessing and as a curse (historically, women always get mixed reviews). And in the moment when the Buddha was enlightened, he was sitting under none other than a fig tree.

In spite of all this suggestive fig subtext, there is no scientific evidence to support the use of figs as an aphrodisiac. We do know that figs have high amounts of antioxidants, flavonoids and polyphenols, though, which are all important for great sex. And that makes figs good enough for us.

If that's not compelling enough, they're an excellent, much healthier sugar substitute, long used to sweeten desserts. You can keep that tradition alive and also toss them into trail mixes and cakes. And best of all, since we're not ashamed of getting naked, we can restrict them to our personal Eden as an appetizer, not a robe of shame.

Garlic *Allium Sativum.*

Even though we all know garlic's true purpose is to kill vampires, that wasn't its original use historically, and also vampires don't exist.

Originating in middle Asia, the use of garlic dates back 5,000 years to Mesopotamia. It may be a culinary mainstay among sophisticated cooks these days, but it was first associated with peasants and laborers. Classism is clearly part smell-ism, and the upper classes of yore thought they were too good to be associated with anything so pungent. The joke was on them, and *The Kamasutra*, the sexual *Pitchfork Review* of its day, was quick on the garlic uptake as a cool aphrodisiac.

They weren't the only ones: Hebrew grooms hung it on marital beds to ensure copulation on the wedding night. Hindu holy men were *forbidden* from eating garlic, lest it inspire dirty lust in their clean minds.[347]

Funnily enough, this is all about antioxidants, of which garlic always lands a perfect score. We know that antioxidants contribute to great sex. They *also* contribute to great balls. Like dates, they increase testicular weight, in this case in as little as three months.[348] Garlic is hot for females too, demonstrating in research the ability to help their cardiovascular system and increase nitric oxide availability.

Big balls. Increased wetness. That's garlic. (Call the Garlic Industry. I think we've got a new slogan.)

Ginger *Zingiber officinale.*

Would you believe that at one point in history you could trade a pound of ginger for a whole sheep? Don't worry, I won't go there.

Where I will go is to Southeast Asia, where this hot spice originated. It's got such staying power that it's been traded for over a thousand years. It's responsible for the existence of the gingerbread man, or rather, Queen Elizabeth I is, who is said to have invented the celebrated tradition. Ireland heard about that and did one better, giving us ginger ale in the 1800s.

The Chinese, as always, knew what was up with ginger, using it extensively in traditional Chinese herbal medicine for its abundant antioxidants and minerals. If you've ever had nausea, vomiting or digestive issues, you know what's up with ginger too.

It not only soothes the stomach (and gets you a whole sheep), but studies have shown safety at reasonable consumption levels and increased sperm count and motility.[349] It also raises testosterone levels.[350]

I'll take ginger any way I can get it, but I highly recommend two easy ways to get more: many Indian dishes, and drinking ginger tonic (I make my own). Ginger tonic is made with ginger, lemon or lime and honey, which is then covered in mineral water. You can make it at home, too, and that way, the sheep is nobody's business.

Nutmeg *Myristica Fragrans.*

If whole sheep aren't your thing, then consider that nutmeg was, at one time, worth its weight in gold.

Nutmeg is a prized spice used for at least the last 3,500 years. In its early history, it grew only among the volcanic islands of Indonesia, which is where that whole weight-in-gold thing happened. In the middle ages, wealthy Europeans bought nutmeg for its medicinal properties (they must've had enough gold). Romans used it as incense. (Because they're Romans.)

Point of fact: It made the Dutch crazy. In 1621, all hopped up on nutmeg, they massacred almost all of the natives in the Banda islands, then enslaved the remaining 1,000, forcing them to work in nutmeg groves. All just to get their greedy hands on the nutmeg.

Americans were just as obsessed with the stuff. Nutmeg was so valuable in early American history, that "nutmeggers" would whittle fake nutmeg out of wood and sell it. This is beginning to sound like nutmeg is the cocaine of spices, but that can't be true, since nutmeg is used in traditional Chinese medicine to help diarrhea, not cause it.

Nutmeg was, of course, another immediately on the radar of *The Kamasutra*, who after all that craziness about nutmeg everywhere else in the world, could not possibly risk his reputation as an expert sex person and not endorse it as an aphrodisiac. Unani medicine, which is also practiced in India, and derived from medieval Muslim physicians of Byzantine Greece, uses this spice to treat sexual disorders.

So what in nutmeg's name is nutmeg doing to us? Studies tell us that people who eat nutmeg turn right around, rush right out, forgetting their wallet and keys, and have more sex.[351] Animals who dip into a little nutmeg on the DL not only get right down to doing it, but they do it better (really hard to imagine how scientists measure "sexual performance" in animals, but okay!) and these animals also do it more often (fun job, scientists!) and with more lust (perhaps the animals fill out a survey afterward). [352]

At this point, if there's anything else you need to know about nutmeg other than to not just drop everything and get a hold of some, I don't think I can help you.

Onion *Allium cepa*.

In biblical times, the people of northern Sinai were happy to live there because, instead of the mantra *location, location, location* for their real estate choices, their list was more like figs, apples and onions. That's a pretty impressive listing for a much maligned vegetable.

Like garlic, the onion is another situation where the more pungent, the better the pumping (sorry). Ancient texts from India, Greece and Egypt describe onions as a powerful sexual aphrodisiac. In medieval Europe, newlyweds would traditionally eat onions on the morning after their wedding night (obviously not before the wedding night, that was garlic time).

And also like garlic, proof of onion's potency is that it's yet another pungent food people were really invested in keeping from a holy man. In Ancient Egypt, celibate priests were forbidden to eat onions, for fear that they would arouse the horny within.

It makes sense, then, that onion raises testosterone in research, but it does so in a few key ways we've been reiterating throughout here for a great sex diet. Eat an onion and your reward is more nitric oxide, which dilates those blood vessels (ahem, wetness, stiffer boner). You'll get boosted hormones that reduce oxidative stress on reproductive structures too. And, you'll see improved insulin sensitivity[353] which is another premium amenity for improved sexual function. (Of note: Chinese garlic chives are in the onion family, and, they too, increase testosterone and antioxidant capacity to improve sexual function.)

Oysters.

Like figs, oysters have always been on the short list of aphrodisiacs, and it goes back to the original player. In the 1700s, the famous Casanova is rumored to have regularly eaten raw oysters for breakfast to boost his libido. In his famous memoir, he recounts the 100 plus women he seduced thanks to oysters (I do hope he thanked them). Oysters are high in our old pal zinc, which lowers cortisol and raises testosterone, and also high in magnesium.

While only limited studies show that oysters induced sexual desire and enhance sexual behavior,[354] I'm think we're all good with Casanova on this one.

Pomegranate *Punica granatum.*

Depending on how you look at it, pomegranates are either an extremely wiley, confusing aphrodisiac or potentially the greatest aphrodisiac on earth.

For instance, legend has it that drops from the bleeding penis of the lustful god Acdestis formed the red pomegranate, which is not an appealing story. A hornier version is that Aphrodite planted the tree, and she was perpetually horny, as you may recall.

As such, Ancient Greeks regarded pomegranates as the symbol for Aphrodite's sensuality, and here, the crimson red seeds are associated with fertility and eroticism, two things we can get behind a lot easier than a bleeding penis.

But back to the dark side, Hades, the god of the underworld, used pomegranate seeds to seduce Persephone, ultimately binding her to him in Hell. That's also not an outcome we're looking for.

Judaism seems to get it right: They associated pomegranates with marriage and fertility for thousands of years, even using the fruit to make wine. Ancient Egyptian hieroglyphs drew pictures of pomegranate trees, indicating they at least knew something was afoot. Babylonians were clearly pomegranate's biggest fan, once ceremoniously sacrificing 500 pomegranates and dates to the goddess Ishtar (finally, not actual humans for once).

Pomegranates, you must've guessed, are loaded with antioxidants,[355] which means they support all three physical systems involved in sexual function: the nervous, endocrine and cardiovascular systems.

The research here matches the fruit's robustness: They improve erectile dysfunction in diabetics by reducing oxidative stress,[356] they protect the vascular system from damage,[357] increasing that good blood-to-the-penis situation (not the bad Acdestis kind that comes *out* of the penis).

Pomegranates wear many hats too: In a study of subjects with enlarged prostates, pomegranate significantly reduced that enlargement.[358] They protect against damage from environmental toxins,[359] and pomegranate extract improves ED caused by damaged arteries.[360]

So in spite of their mixed mythological reputation, thanks to modern science, we can finally trust them.

Prunes *Prunus domestica.*

I can be sure you're not expecting this sentence, but brothels in 16th century England served up prunes to get their customers horny. (I have a lot of questions too).

No scientific evidence supports the use of prunes as an aphrodisiac, though, and there's also the whole prunes-for-constipation thing that seems counter to our goals here.

That said, for my money, a brothel is a female-run business, and I support female-run businesses, and so should you. We need more of them. In this case, that business needed horny customers, so they went with prunes. Think about it.

Saffron *Crocus sativus.*

If you're like me, the first thing you think of when you think about saffron is holy smokes, why is saffron so expensive? Is it the dust of golden silk spun by a mythical spider?

No, it's just extremely laborious to cultivate. Saffron is the stamen of the saffron crocus, which is in the iris family. Many of these tiny stamen must be harvested in order to make a small amount of saffron. For this reason, saffron is among the most expensive spices in the world.

At least with saffron we find one of the most scientifically studied plant aphrodisiacs, and it delivers. The active constituent, crocin, was found in research to increase libido,[361] frequency of erections, post ejaculatory copulation and improve ease of erections.[362] It was also found to improve arousal, lubrication and decrease vaginal pain in women suffering from depression.[363]

Saffron has been shown clinically to have cardio-protective properties, reducing blood pressure, preventing clotting, reducing cholesterol, protecting against atherosclerosis and serving as a vasodilator, bringing blood to the genitals. It also brings more oxygen to tissues,[364] which enhances performance.[365]

So basically, saffron means better sex with less work. You can't put a price on that.

Sweet potato *Ipomoea batatas.*

Quick, what food instantly makes you think bodily lust? If you didn't say sweet potato, have I got news for you.

In 1597, John Gerard of England wrote in *Herball or Generall Historie of Plantes*, that sweet potatoes "procured bodily lust," and they were quite popular among upper class during this time.

In research, sweet potato impressed the judges with its aphrodisiac score, and in its protective effect on sex organs in male subjects. Sweet potato significantly increased sexual desire, improved sperm health, positively affected sex hormones, including levels of testosterone, LH, FSH and estradiol. Additionally, it protected against damage from environmental toxins (such as BPA, found in plastics).[366]

Originating in Latin America, sweet potato root is now a staple in the world diet and should also be a staple in the sex diet.

Tamarind *Tamarindus indica.*

Nothing says sexy like a food you can eat, take as medicine or use to polish metal. But that's tamarind for you, an aphrodisiac that doubles as a lusty metal worker's dream. It's technically a tree native to tropical Africa with bean-like pods that make a thick dark paste that is used in all the above.

It's also widely used in Indian, Mexican, Malaysian and other cuisines. As early as 400 BCE, this fruit was already consumed in Egypt and Greece.

In Latin America, tamarind is used to make the drink *agua de tamarindo*. In Indian cooking it is used to flavor chutneys and sauces. Try butter chicken drizzled with a bit of tamarind sauce, as it adds a bit of tart sweetness to it. Also, if you ever make your own barbecue sauce, tamarind can be the secret ingredient that adds the perfect sweet acidity.

Tamarind may not come to mind when you think "sex food," but it gets the job done, and easily through foods you likely already eat or should now be motivated to try. It's rich in calcium, phosphorus, iron, thiamine, niacin and riboflavin. Sperm motility and sperm count significantly increased with use of tamarind, as did sexual arousal and desire.[367] In another study,[368] tamarind made a small but statistically significant improvement in premature ejaculation in men.

Thai black ginger *Kaempferia parviflora.*

Thai black ginger does not only enhance male sexual function in bed but also in Thai martial arts. Also known as Thai ginseng, it's native to Bangladesh, Cambodia, Myanmar and Thailand.

In research, Thai black ginger did all the things and did them well: improved blood flow to the genitals, sexual frequency and ease of ejaculation.[369] It also improved sexual response to erotic stimuli.[370] In other studies it improved energy metabolism for improved physical performance and muscle endurance.[371]

If you're the sort of person who loves food, sex *and* martial arts, put Thai black ginger on your list.

Vanilla *Vanilla planifolia.*

Vanilla is usually the last thing you want your sex to be, although I think vanilla gets a bad rep. Remember back when we chatted about the Aztecs mixing vanilla and chocolate together? That tidbit came from Hernán Cortés in the 1500s, who brought loads of both of these luscious treats back to Spain as souvenirs (he skipped the human sacrifice).

Cut to the 1800s and doctors are recommending vanilla prior to sexual activity to stimulate arousal. While I found no studies to test this reputation, let's not undercut vanilla's history, nor its gift to the taste buds on our quest for sensual pleasure.

Wood ear mushrooms *Auricularia polytricha.*

You thought you were done hearing about mushrooms, but alas, we meet again. Relax, I'm just here to sing the praises of one special species out of the whole 50,000. The wood ear. Hey, the wood part sounds good!

Also known as black fungus, wood ear mushrooms are found all over the world and have been used for millennia as food and medicine. In traditional Chinese medicine, they are known to nourish the yin and benefit the cardiovascular and immune systems.

Research has demonstrated that wood ear mushrooms are potent aphrodisiacs,[372] increasing sexual behavior and ejaculation in male mice. In research, these mushrooms helped subjects overcome stress-induced sexual dysfunction, improving desire, ease of orgasm and probability of post-ejaculatory sexual desire. So let's be happy for those mice and consider adding wood ear to any soup recipe to get in on this party.

Medicinal Substances

Below are some medicinals that have been studied for aphrodisiac effect. Consider this informational a guide for exploration with an expert. While I emphatically do not recommend self-prescribing these substances, as it would be like prescribing oneself prescription drugs, I do recommend determining the therapeutic and safe dosage with a qualified practitioner who has an extensive knowledge of herbal medicine.

Not only can they guide you to which substances you need, but experts are better at recognizing adverse reactions, duration of treatment and other considerations. They should also help manage expectations for you, telling you how long before you can expect to see results and how long prior to sex should you take the substance.

Ashwagandha *Withania somnifera.*
Want the endurance of a horse in bed? Who doesn't? This herb's use in Ayurveda dates back thousands of years. It is classified as Vaji-karana, which means that it promotes healthy sexual functioning. *The Kamasutra* also recommends ashwagandha as an aphrodisiac, believing it confers the strength and stamina of a horse and increases fertility. Many African tribes use ashwagandha for inflammation and fevers.

Research[373] suggests that ashwaganda is safe and effective to improve sexual function in women[374] and in men.[375] Ashwaghanda increased DHEA and testosterone in older overweight subjects.[376] Further-more, it increased sperm count, semen volume and motility in men with low sperm count.[377]

Astragalus *Radix astragali.*
Astragalus is known in traditional Chinese medicine as huang qi, or yellow qi, because its root is yellowish and it supports the qi. In research, astragalus increased sperm counts[378] and motility.[379]

Bufo toad *Rhinella marina.*
One of the more unusual aphrodisiacs, also known as the Love Stone, this substance is found in the skin glands of the Bufo toad. Research demonstrated that the risks of this potentially toxic substance outweigh the benefits.[380]

Burdock root *Arctium lappa L.*
Abundant in flavonoids, saponins, lignans and alkaloids, burdock root was found in research to enhance sexual behavior and performance.[381]

Chione venosa.
The stem, bark and roots of this plant are harvested from the Carib-bean island of Grenada. Studies found that the chemical composi-tion of this plant made it an effective aphrodisiac.[382]

Chrysactinia *Chrysactinia mexicana.*
Also called "False Damiana," this plant, native to Mexico and the Southwestern US, stimulated sexual activity in clinical studies. It

enhanced sexual performance and improved ability to ejaculate without delay.

Cihuapatli *Montanoa tomentosa.*
This plant demonstrated aphrodisiac properties in research, increasing libido, and promoted masculine sexual behavior in those who were sexually inactive.[383]

Cordyceps *Ophiocordyceps sinensis.*
Cordyceps enhances the way our cells use oxygen, boosting both energy and performance. With 2,000 years of use in China for great sex, it's antiviral and lands in *The Kamasutra.*

As noted in the mushroom chapter, it has measurable improvements in libido and desire in both men and women, increases testosterone in males and significantly improves sperm count and sperm quality.[384]

Cordyceps also protects against oxidative stress,[385] benefits cholesterol and lowers triglycerides. It is a natural vasodilator, which increases blood flow to sex organs.

Chuan Xiong *Ligusticum Chuanxiong.*
Moves the qi to move the blood. In research it was shown to increase cyclic guanosine monophosphate (cGMP) and cyclic adenosine monophosphate (cAMP).[386]

Cynomorii *Herba Cynomorii.*
This fleshy stem is called suo yang in traditional Chinese medicine. Country women used to use this herb internally as an aphrodisiac, and also as a natural dildo, by inserting it into their vagina, which swells as it absorbs vaginal secretions.[387]

Damiana *Turnera diffusa.*
In the same family as the passion flower, the leaves of this plant are used in folk medicine as an aphrodisiac, pain reliever and for anti-anxiety.[388] It makes male subjects want to have sex, even when they are sexually exhausted,[389] after having had plenty of sex already. It's anyone's guess why this isn't in every rom-com, salon and retail outlet, but we can dream. This effect was probably related to its high antioxidant levels, immune-boosting and anti-microbial properties.[390]

Damiana also demonstrated a positive affect on testosterone,[391] and positively impacted estrogen, which is involved in male and female arousal. Damiana works by increasing the availability of nitric oxide in the body.[392]

Convulsions and symptoms similar to rabies have been reported at higher doses, though, so buyer beware.

Ginko leaves *Folium Bilobae.*

In research it was shown to increase nitric oxide synthase expression and dopaminergic activity.[393]

Ginseng *Radix ginseng.*

Ginseng has a reputation across Asia as an effective aphrodisiac. It was used to stimulate the sexual appetite and also in the management of erectile dysfunction as early as 3500 BCE. Ancient texts state that "Ginseng strengthens the soul, brightens the eyes, opens the heart, expels evil, benefits understanding, and if taken for prolonged periods of time will invigorate the body and prolong one's life."[394]

While that leaves it unclear if it's an aphrodisiac or a cult, I can tell you that in studies, ginseng was found to have antioxidant properties and induced erections.[395]

Horny goat weed *Epimedii herba.*

Hooboy, now we're talking. In traditional Chinese medicine this herb is called yin yang huo and is used as a treatment in sexual dysfunction due to its vasodilatory effect.[396]

Studies have shown that horny goat weed is an aptly named substance that restores low levels of testosterone and thyroid hormones closer to normal levels. However, there is potential toxicity with using this substance, so maybe it should be called "horny potentially dangerous goat weed."

Human placenta *Hominis placenta.*

Unless you're already down with the placenta situation, this might sound strange as an edible, but bear with me. In traditional Chinese medicine, this substance is called zi he che and is used for infertility, impotence, spermatorrhea and decreased libido.

For women, pregnancy and delivery taxes the qi, blood and depletes the essence. Human placenta is believed to augment this essence, which is why a common practice is for a mother to cook and eat her placenta after birth (I'm sure you've come across a celebrity or two talking about it).

But it's not just celebrities and woo-woo types. I have known some of my acupuncturist friends to do this, just in case you didn't think we were weird enough already.

Maca *Lepidium meyenii.*
Maca grows in the Peruvian Andes and is used traditionally as an aphrodisiac and to enhance fertility. In research, Maca improved sexual desire,[397] erectile function and performance. It decreased the time it took for subjects to become erect and increased libido.[398] In other studies, Maca improved female sexual function.[399]

Make maca your friend.

Rou Cong Rong *Herba cistanche.*
In TCM, Rou Cong Rong is known to nourish kidney yang. In research it was shown to increase testosterone levels.[400]

San Qi *Radix notoginseng.*
San Qi moves the blood. In research it was shown to reduce oxidative stress and increase NOS expression.[401]

Schisandra fruit *Schisandra chinensis.*
Schisandra causes relaxation of vascular smooth muscle. Studies showed that it helped Viagra to work more effectively.[402] I say skip the Viagra first and try it by itself.

Spanish fly *Lytta vesicatoria.*
Spanish fly, long the punchline in cartoonish portrayals of desire, is in fact a real substance and not just a lazy plot device. Perhaps no aphrodisiac on earth is more invoked and more misunderstood. Such creative portrayals and folklore have effectively muddled the myth, and Spanish fly should be approached with extreme caution.

First, what it is: Spanish fly is made from blister beetles, which produce the active substance cantharidin. While it appears that this aphrodisiac does promote erection by irritating the urogenital tract, leading to excessive blood flow to the genitals, it may also lead to priapism, a painful, persistent erection that goes on long after you're done.

And it must be noted: There have been countless fatalities from the use of Spanish fly throughout the ages,[403] not to mention lots of devious horsin' around with it.

Spanish fly is still used to encourage breeding in animals today, but most available medical literature describes Spanish fly as not only unreliable but with a very thin margin between effective and toxic doses. Most studies found that the risks of this substance far outweigh the benefits.[404] In minor reactions, it can cause painful urination, bloody stools and vomiting, and more seriously causes kidney and liver damage, which may lead to death. Try getting a seduction on with those problems.

When there are dozens of other options here, let's just leave Spanish fly to Hollywood, where they can undoubtedly have a lot more fun giving it to fictional characters.

Tu Si Zi *Semen cuscutae.*
In TCM, Tu Si Zi is understood to nourish kidney yin, yang and jing. In research it was shown to increase testosterone levels.[405]

Tribulus *Tribuli fructus.*
Tribulus is known as ci ji li in traditional Chinese medicine, and Gokshura in Ayurvedic medicine. Caltrop, cat's head and bindii are all common names of this plant.

Though this substance can be toxic in higher doses, toxicity studies suggested that it was safe at lower doses. In research, the fruit improves erectile strength and ejaculation, increases desire and significantly increases testosterone in both younger and older males.[406] Tribulus increases testosterone, improves erections and also sperm count.[407] In traditional Iranian medicine it is used in combination with anacyclus pyrethrum to effectively improve fertility.[408]

For female sexual dysfunction, Tribulus was found to be both safe and effective in clinical research. In one study, 250 females with sexual dysfunction were given tribulus daily for ninety days. Eighty-eight percent experienced improvement. In several studies, women had a statistically significant increase in desire, arousal, orgasm, satisfaction[409] and lubrication.[410]

Yohimbine *Pausinystalia johimbe.*

The bark of Yohimbe trees is a common aphrodisiac in West Africa and one with higher potential for toxicity.

Derived from those trees, Yohimbine is approved for use by the FDA. It stimulates the pelvic nerve ganglia and boosts adrenaline supply to nerve endings. It also works by dilating blood vessels, increasing blood flow to the genitals. For this reason, it would likely be useful for females as well. It effectively treated men who had difficulty achieving orgasm.[411] One review, however, found that the risks of this substance outweigh the benefits.[412]

PART IV:
THE FUN PART:
PRACTICING WHAT
YOU'VE LEARNED

GREAT SEX ACTION PLAN

We've discussed how to think differently about sex, about how our bodies experience pleasure, how our minds are equally integral to the process, and how the history of traditional Chinese medicine, through acupuncture, diet and philosophy, form the underpinnings of this approach.

Now, we need an action plan to bring it all together.

How to Eat Your Way to Horny

For the holy trinity of great sex—improved nerve signaling to and from the genitals, balanced sex hormones and better blood flow—do the following:

Limit

- Fats such as fried foods, many baked goods, fatty meats, oils
- Processed foods such as chips, fast food, canned and boxed foods that you can
  barely tell what they were in nature
- Salty foods such as processed meals, fast food and salt added in cooking
- Refined sugars such as baked goods, candy, sweets, drinks with added sugars,
  and sodas
- Refined grains such as white rice, white pasta and most bread
- Rich, heavy foods that slow the qi like dairy, pork and processed meats

Increase

Antioxidants	Fruits and vegetables, especially leafy greens, and berries, as well as mushrooms contain antioxidants such as the following: • Polyphenols • Vitamin C • Vitamin A • Vitamin E
Micronutrients	• B-Vitamins: which are found in fruits and vegetables, nuts and seeds • Naturally nitrate-rich foods including leafy greens and vegetables like beets, celery, cabbage and radish • Potassium-rich foods including banana, squash, potato, yam, mango, leafy greens, oranges, cantaloupe, figs, kiwi, avocado and broccoli • Calcium, magnesium, zinc and other minerals, which are found in nuts, fruits, vegetables and especially leafy greens • Brassica vegetables like broccoli, cauliflower, kale, Brussels sprouts, arugula, cabbage, radish and collard greens • Leafy greens every day such as spinach, arugula, green leaf lettuce, red leaf lettuce and romaine • Omega 3 fatty acid-rich foods such as fish, flax seeds and walnuts
Get Adequate Sunlight	Just 10 to 30 minutes in midday sun
Exercise Daily	Even if you can't get to the gym, all you need to do is move more in your own environment. • Take a walk on your lunch break • Hit the stairs for 15 minutes • Bike to the store or to run errands • Get crazy in bed
Do a gentle fast weekly (See chapter 2)	

1-Week Sample Menu

	Day 1	Day 2	Day 3
Breakfast	Fruit: try to include at least half of a banana, mango or orange. If you need more food, add oatmeal, no butter or fat	3 Ingredient Banana Pancakes (recipe on page 172)	Fruit: try to include at least half of a banana, mango or orange. If you need more food, add oatmeal, no butter or fat
Snack	1 handful of walnuts	1 handful of cashews	1 handful of almonds
Lunch	Spinach salad with broccoli, celery, onions and tomatoes. Top with vinaigrette dressing (recipe on page 174)	Romaine salad with shredded red cabbage, cucumber and carrots, toasted pecans. Add ranch dressing (recipe on page 176)	Green leaf salad with red peppers, cauliflower, parsley, avocado, sprouts. Add creamy balsamic dressing (recipe on page 175)
	Baked potato with pepper and a pinch of salt	Sliced mango	Steamed vegetable of your choice
Dinner	Pan-seared Wild Salmon (recipe on page 183). Steamed asparagus, Roasted Spiced Squash (recipe on page 184)	Mushroom Sofrias burrito bowls (recipe on page 181) topped with fresh salsa and guacamole (recipe on page 190)	Lentils cooked with onions, carrots, cauliflower, potato and tomato with curry, served over potato or yam
Snack	Sliced apples with cinnamon	Berries topped with coconut yogurt and sprinked with roasted pecans	Celery and carrots with hummus

Day 4	Day 5	Day 6	Day 7
Go-to Green Smoothie (recipe on page 171)	Fruit: try to include at least half of a banana, mango or orange. If you need more food, add oatmeal, no butter or fat	Fruit with Emily's Granola (recipe on page 173)	Fruit: try to include at least half of a banana, mango or orange. If you need more food, add oatmeal, no butter or fat
1 handful of pecans	1 handful of mixed nuts	1 handful of pistachios	1 handful of sunflower seeds
Arugula and mixed green salad with red onion, veggies of choice and steamed beets. Top with vinaigrette dressing (recipe on page 174)	Green leaf salad with steamed brussels sprouts, purple carrots and veggies of choice. Add ranch dressing (recipe on page 176)	Mixed green salad with chopped kale, veggies of choice, steamed asparagus and avocado. Add creamy balsamic dressing (recipe on page 175)	Butter leaf lettuce with radishes, sliced mushrooms and purple cauliflower. Add vinaigrette dressing (recipe on page 174)
Sliced cantaloupe	Baked yam with pepper and a pinch of salt	Sliced kiwi with figs	Pan-seared summer squash with pepper, thyme and a pinch of salt
Mushroom Makhani (recipe on page 179)	Tuscan Kale Soup (recipe on page 185) with steamed cod	Pesto Noodles (recipe on page 178) with Butternut Squash Soup (recipe on page 186)	Beans and rice of your choice served with plantains and Nicaraguan Cabbage Salad (recipe on page 177).
Mangonada (recipe on page 196)	Pink Fluffy Nice Cream (recipe on page 192)	Sliced pears sprinkled with cinnamon	Sliced oranges

Pre-Game Eating for a Hot Date

Some foods have an immediate effect on blood vessels, for better or worse.

Avoid, Day-Of

- High fat
- Salt

Encourage All Day

Potassium-rich, nitrate rich and flavonoid-rich foods have been shown in research to have an immediately (within two hours) positive effect on blood vessels. The magnitude of this effect has not been well studied and is generally subtle yet significant enough to be measured.

For the best sex, long-term healthy eating is the best strategy. You can combine these foods with some of the aphrodisiac foods and spices we've discussed. Below are some guidelines for creating a date-night sex menu for a night of hot sex.

Date Night Sex Menu

Eat	Why
Salad	
Leafy greens such as spinach, green leaf lettuce, romaine, parsley, cilatro etc.	After you eat nitrate rich vegetables, nitric oxide levels increase in your body, peaking about two hours after eating. Nitric oxide dilates blood vessels, which affects sexual arousal and pleasure. Leafy greens also make blood vessels more pliable, further improving delivery of oxygen-rich blood to the clitoris, vagina and penis.
Beets, celery, radish, red cabbage, fennel	These vegetables are also rich in nitrates. See above.
Onions, kale, broccoli, celery	Rich in flavonoids. Flavonoid-rich foods make blood vessels more elastic very shortly after eating.
Cruciferous vegetables such as broccoli, cauliflower, cabbage, kale, brussels sprouts, arugula	Brassica vegetables contain numerous phyto-nutrients that have been shown in research to benefit sexual function for males and females.

Potassium-rich foods	
Potato, yam, squash, orange, banana, mango	Potassium-rich foods make blood vessels more pliable and increase nitric oxide release shortly after eating. Lasting for several hours.
Omega 3s	
Wild salmon: 3-4 oz	Omega 3s improve vascular function for increased bloodflow and increased pleasure.
Walnuts: 1 small handful	See above.
Polyphenols	
Cherries, onions, apples, berries, kale, leeks, broccoli, blueberries, parsley, fresh citrus fruits, celery	Polyphenols measurably improve vascular function within hours of eating.
Aphrodisiac foods	
Cloves, Saffron, nutmeg, onions, chile peppers, dates, dill, fennel, fenugreek, garlic, ginger, tamarind, wood ear mushrooms. See chapter 13 for more.	All of these culinary aphrodisiacs have demonstrated in research the ability to improve sexual function or pleasure. Some, such as cloves, improve desire and performance in as little as an hour after eating them.

Avoid	Why
Fatty foods	A fatty meal makes blood vessels measurably stiffer within a couple hours. More pliable blood vessels are able to deliver more blood to the clitoris, vagina and penis. More blood means more pleasure and better performance.
Salty foods	Research has shown that blood vessels are measurably stiffer within thirty minutes of eating a salty meal, reducing nitric oxide release.

Don't Forget to Focus on Them

Any plan for great sex must include action to broaden our efforts beyond our natural selfishness, to nourish kindness toward our partner. Kindness can take on different forms, but in the bedroom, it means taking the time and effort to learn how to care for our partner sexually. When we regard our partner as an equal, we realize that we must focus on their sexual pleasure as much as our own. When both yin and yang are happy, sex is harmoniously delightful.

Sex Partner Activity

This is an activity to both communicate your sexual needs with your partner, and also to help you to be a kinder lover, thinking beyond your own pleasure. Sure, it might feel a little cheesy at first, but the result will be hot sex.

1. How can I/do I care for my partner in bed?

_____

_____

_____

2. How can I/do I care for my partner out of bed?

_____

_____

_____

3. I try to please my partner less than / as much as / more than I try to please myself in bed. Out of bed?

_____

_____

_____

4. How would I like my partner to care for me?

_____

_____

_____

5. What do I like about my partner's touch?

_____

_____

_____

6. What would I like more of?

_____

_____

_____

7. It doesn't work for me when my partner…

_____

_____

_____

8. When my partner touches me, or stimulates me sexually, the pressure/stimulation is (circle all that apply)

often too light   often too heavy   often just right   almost always just right

9. What do I want my partner to add next time?

_____

_____

_____

10. It would be really hot if we…

_____

_____

_____

Diet for Great Sex Daily Planner

Here's an organizational tool to keep you on track with your diet for great sex:

Date:_____

Breakfast:

_____

_____

Lunch:

_____

_____

Dinner:

_____

_____

Snack:

_____

_____

Did you include enough of these?

☐	Antioxidants
☐	Mushrooms
☐	Fruits
☐	Vegetables
☐	Leafy Greens
☐	Cruciferous veggies
☐	Potassium-rich foods
☐	Omega 3s
☐	Nuts
☐	Sunlight
☐	Hydration

Exercise:

Activity: _____ Duration: _____

Activity: _____ Duration: _____

Activity: _____ Duration: _____

Acts of kindness toward my partner:

_____

_____

Had sex today? Notes:

_____

_____

Recipes

Here are some great recipes, most developed by Emily Daniels, of Wholesome Hedonista. http://www.wholesomehedonista.com. Emily is a genius in the kitchen and can take any dietary guidelines and create absolutely delicious food. You can view videos of the recipes at @wholesomehedonista on Instagram.

Sex Smoothie

This pre-sex smoothie recipe has potassium-rich banana as well as poly-phenol-rich blueberries and nitrate-rich spinach as well as aphrodisiac ginger, maca and saffron. This tasty smoothie makes for blood vessels that deliver optimal flow to our genitals.

Prep Time	Cook Time
5 min	0

Course	Breakfast/snack
Serves	1

Ingredients

1.5 cups frozen blueberries
1 cup spinach (packed)
1 banana
1 Tbsp minced/grated ginger
1 Tbsp maca powder
A pinch of saffron
1/2 cup to 1 cup water, as needed for desired consistency

Instructions

1. Mix all of the ingredients in a blender or food processor until smooth.

Go-to Green Smoothie

This go-to smoothie recipe has antioxidant and potassium-rich mango and banana as well as nitrate-rich spinach for blood vessels that deliver optimal flow to our genitals, to get the sex flowing.

Prep Time	Cook Time
5 min	0
Course	Breakfast/snack
Serves	1

Ingredients

1 cup spinach
1/2 cup frozen mango
1/2 banana
1/2 lime, squeezed
1/2 cup plant milk or water
Thumb of ginger

Instructions

1. Mix all of the ingredients in a blender or food processor until smooth. Garnish with chia seeds if desired.

Recipe from Emily Daniels at Wholesome Hedonista. For full video, visit: https://www.instagram.com/p/CBTN48rJN0O/

3-Ingredient Banana Pancakes

High in potassium to luxuriate blood vessels leading to the genitals, these pancakes are simple and delicious for luxurious sex.

Prep Time	Cook Time
10 min	8 min

Course	Breakfast/snack
Serves	2

Ingredients

3/4 cup oats
1 and 1/2 ripe bananas
1/3 cup almond milk
Maple syrup

Toppings (optional)

Banana
Pecans
Cinnamon, cloves, nutmeg

Instructions

1. Blend oats in a high-powered blender until fine, like flour.
2. Add bananas and almond milk and a pinch of salt and cinnamon if desired. Blend until smooth.
3. Pour batter onto a non-stick, lightly greased pan and cook until bubbles appear all over, especially the center.
4. Top with your favorite toppings.

Recipe from Emily Daniels at Wholesome Hedonista. For full video, visit: https://www.instagram.com/p/CAqTLGPpF-k/

Emily's Granola

What's more 'granola' than regular granola? An oil-free, grain-fee granola. This pumpkin spice granola has a hearty crunchiness with aphrodisiac cloves and nutmeg to add spice to your sex life. The walnuts also offer amazing sex benefits with their antioxidants and omega 3s.

Prep Time	Cook Time
20 min	20 min
Course	Breakfast
Serves	6

Ingredients

1 cup raw walnuts
1/2 cup raw slivered or sliced almonds
1/2 cup raw pumpkin seeds
3 Tbsp raw hemp seeds
1/2 cup chopped dates
1/2 cup coconut flakes
1/4 tsp ground cloves
1/2 tsp ground nutmeg
1/2 cup pure maple syrup
1/2 cup almond butter, salted
1 tsp pure vanilla extract

Instructions

1. Preheat oven to 325°F and place rack in center position.
2. Stir together all ingredients in a large bowl until well combined.
3. Spread in a thin layer on a baking sheet lined with parchment paper.
4. Bake for 15-20 minutes, turning once or twice. Longer for crispier. Store in an airtight container for up to a few weeks.
5. Serve over fresh fruit such as berries and bananas.

Recipe from Emily Daniels at Wholesome Hedonista. For full video, visit: https://www.instagram.com/p/B5LFApWFrQk/

The Best Oil-free Vinaigrette Ever!

This dressing is loaded with flavor to make your lunchtime sex salad (and sex) delicious!

Prep Time	Cook Time
15 min	0
Course	Lunch/Dinner
Serves	6

Ingredients

1 small/medium onion, finely chopped
2-3 lemons, juiced
2 cloves garlic minced
1 big handful of your favorite fresh herbs like dill or basil
1/4-1/2 tsp black pepper (I like to put a lot in)
A pinch of salt. More tastes better, but less is best for great sex
A drizzle of olive oil (Only if you want. It tastes great without it.)

Organic leafy greens and veggies of your choice. Be sure to include cruciferous like broccoli or cauliflower.

Instructions

1. Chop onions and herbs finely
2. Juice lemons or limes
3. Mix ingredients together. You may add a small amount of olive oil, but it tastes great without it. Less is better.
4. Serve over a green salad of your choice.

Oil-free Creamy Balsamic Dressing

Leafy greens are probably the best food in existence for great sex, so it's essential to have a lot of delicious options for dressing them. This balsamic is out of this world (like the sex you'll soon be having).

Prep Time	Cook Time
20 min	0
Course	Lunch/Dinner
Serves	6

Ingredients

3/4 cup raw cashews
2/3 cup balsamic vinegar
1 clove garlic
1 tsp mustard, Dijon or regular
1/2 tsp salt
Fresh pepper
2-4 soaked soft dates
1/4 cup water to thin (optional)

Instructions

1. Soak cashews in water for 3 hours.
2. Drain cashews.
3. Blend all ingredients in a high-powered blender until creamy. Add water to thin if needed.

Delicious Nut-based Ranch Dressing

This ranch dressing is loaded with sex-nourishing herbs and culinary aphrodisiacs to cultivate your sex life. It is dairy-free, using zinc-rich cashews as the base.

Prep Time	Cook Time
20 min	0

Course	Lunch/Dinner
Serves	6

Ingredients

1 cup raw cashews, soaked
2-3 cloves garlic
2 soft dates, pitted
Juice of a half lemon or lime
1/2 tsp pepper
Salt to taste (less is always better for sex)
A handful of fresh parsley
A handful of fresh chives
A handful of fresh dill

Instructions

1. Soak cashews overnight. Drain liquid.
2. Blend cashews, garlic, dates, lemon juice, pepper and salt in a blender or food processor. Add a little bit of water if needed for a creamy consistency.
3. Add finely chopped herbs.
4. Serve with leafy greens and vegetables of your choice. For great sex, be sure to include cruciferous vegetables like broccoli or cauliflower.

Nicaraguan Cabbage Salad

This delicious salad contains no oil plus sex-healthy cruciferous vegetables for your big bang. I like to make beans and rice and top it with a big handful of this salad, which adds a zesty fresh flavor. This is how it is served in Nicaragua, over gallo pinto, which is the national red bean and rice dish eaten daily.

Prep Time	Cook Time
20 min	0
Course	Lunch/Dinner
Serves	6

Ingredients

4 cups finely shredded green cabbage
1 cup finely shredded carrot
Juice of 2 limes
1 Tbsp vinegar
2 jalapeños or other chile finely diced
Salt to taste (less is better for great sex)

Instructions

1. Mix chopped jalapeños, salt and lime juice in a small dish. Let sit for 15 minutes.
2. Shred cabbage and carrots.
3. Combine cabbage mixture and lime juice/pepper/salt.
4. Serve over any savory dish like beans and rice.

Pesto Noodles

Sex-happy spinach, basil, walnuts, garlic and avocado make for a delicious noodle dish that will put a smile on your face.

Prep Time	Cook Time
20 min	20 min

Course	Lunch/Dinner
Serves	4

Ingredients

1 cup basil
1 cup spinach
3 tsp raw walnuts
1.5 Tbsp fresh lemon juice
2 cloves garlic
1/2 ripe avocado
1/4 cup water (more if needed)
Salt to taste (less is better for sex)
1/4 tsp pepper
Noodles of choice (kelp, rice, buckwheat or other)

Instructions

1. Boil noodles according to directions.
2. Blend all other ingredients in a blender or food processor.
3. Toss noodles with pesto.
4. Top with your favorite toppings like fresh tomatoes, pine nuts or crushed red pepper.

Mushroom Makhani

This fragrantly spiced Indian dish, also known as Butter Chicken (this recipe uses mushrooms instead), will butter your chicken. This non-dairy, version, sweetened with dates, is a great way to enjoy sex-healthy foods like antioxidant-rich, genital nerve-healthy mushrooms and aphrodisiac spices like black pepper, cloves and nutmeg (in garam masala) as well as fenugreek, garlic and ginger.

Prep Time	Cook Time
20 min	20 min
Course	Dinner
Serves	6

Ingredients

2 pounds mushrooms of your choice
2 Tbsp olive oil
1 large onion, sliced thin
2 tsp garlic, minced
2 tsp ginger, grated or finely shredded
3 cups cherry tomatoes (about 14oz) or 1 14.5 oz can
1 tsp chili powder
1 1/2 tsp coriander powder
1 1/2 tsp ground cumin
10 dates
1 Tbsp tomato paste
3/4 cup canned coconut milk
1/2 tsp garam masala
1/2 tsp fenugreek leaves
2 tsp salt, or to taste
Black pepper to taste

Instructions

1. Heat olive oil in a large skillet over medium heat. Add onions and sautee until soft and translucent. Add ginger and garlic, stir and cook for 30 seconds.
2. Next add tomatoes, dates, chilli powder, coriander and cumin, along with 1/4 cup water. Cook for 5-10 minutes, carefully crushing tomatoes as they heat to release their juices. Stir in tomato paste.
3. Transfer mixture to a blender and blend until completely smooth (you may have to add another 1/4 cup water to blend more easily).
4. Sauté mushrooms in 1 tsp olive oil until browned. Add sauce and heat through. When it starts to bubble, add coconut milk and garam masala.
5. Serve over potato, brown rice or cauliflower rice and sprinkle with chopped cilantro and dried fenugreek leaves

Recipe from Emily Daniels at Wholesome Hedonista. For full video, visit: https://www.instagram.com/p/B764Ggzp7Aw/

Chipotle-inspired Mushroom Sofritas

If you've ever gone to Chipotle and ordered a burrito bowl, then you know what this is. But instead of shredded tofu, we use shredded mushrooms and add in sex-healthy garlic, chiles and cilantro for a kick your sex life won't forget.

Prep Time	Cook Time
20 min	20 min
Course	Lunch/Dinner
Serves	6

Ingredients

1 1/2 pounds mushrooms such as oyster, lion's mane or just plain white
1 roasted poblano pepper
1-3 (depending on your spice preference) canned chipotle peppers in adobo sauce
2 Tbsp reserved adobo sauce
2-3 garlic cloves
2 Tbsp fresh lime juice (about 1 lime)
1 1/2 Tbsp pure maple syrup
1/2 cup salsa (or better yet, use the homemade salsa recipe in this book)
1/2 jalapeño pepper finely diced
1/4 cup cilantro
1 tsp salt and pepper to taste
1 Tbsp olive oil (optional)
Avocado for garnish

Instructions

1. Add all ingredients except mushrooms, avocado and oil to the food processor and blend on high until smooth. Set this sauce aside.
2. Shred mushrooms with a cheese shredder or food processor.
3. In a large non-stick pan heat oil (or omit for oil-free). Cook mushrooms until some of the water cooks off.

4. Mix in sofritas sauce and cook for about 10 minutes.
5. Serve over rice or cauliflower rice and garnish with cilantro, avocado and lime.

Recipe from Emily Daniels at Wholesome Hedonista. For full video, visit: https://www.instagram.com/p/B8RyMdbpONq/

Pan-seared Wild Salmon with Herbs

If you're going to include fish in your diet for their abundant omega-3 fatty acids, you have to have a great basic wild salmon recipe. Omega 3s help nerves fire more quickly and strongly to and from the genitals. They also improve function of blood vessels which carry blood to where we need it most during hot sex.

Prep Time	Cook Time
5 min	10 min
Course	Lunch/Dinner
Serves	2

Ingredients

2 salmon filets, rinsed, patted dry with paper towel
1 tsp butter or coconut oil
A few sprigs of any fresh herbs that you like. Thyme works really well!
Salt and pepper to taste (less salt is better for sex)
1 tsp soy sauce (or omit for lower salt)

Instructions

1. Take out the salmon 20 minutes prior to cooking. Make sure you pat it dry. This will make for moister fish. If you have time, dry age it a bit longer by leaving it overnight uncovered in the fridge, seasoned with just a bit of salt and pepper.
2. Heat butter/coconut oil in a non-stick skillet at medium to medium-high heat.
3. When the oil is hot, place salmon filets skin-side-down in the pan. Add fresh herbs to the pan for flavor. Cook until the pink flesh just starts to lighten at the bottom, usually just a few minutes, then flip.
4. Add 1 tsp soy sauce to the pan. Cook an additional 2 minutes, until there is a beautiful caramel glaze on your salmon. You can omit the soy sauce to keep salt even lower.
5. Serve with your choice of vegetables, such as yams and asparagus.

Roasted Spiced Squash

This squash is filling, delicious and loaded with sex-healthy potassium and antioxidants. In addition, this recipe contains the aphrodisiac spices cloves and nutmeg for a sweet and savory sex food.

Prep Time	Cook Time
10 min	50 min
Course	Dinner
Serves	2-4

Ingredients

1 acorn or other winter squash
A sprinkle of cinnamon
A sprinkle of nutmeg
A very small sprinkle of ground cloves
Pepper to taste

Instructions

1. Preheat the oven to 350°F. Halve the squash, remove seeds and place on a baking sheet.
2. Sprinkle spices on squash and add a few tablespoons of water to the center hollow of the squash.
3. Bake for about 50 minutes. Check that the squash is very soft and tender.

Tuscan Kale Potato Soup

This delicious recipe contains all the sexual benefits of the nitrate-rich brassica vegetable kale as well as potassium-rich potatoes for flexible healthy arteries, not to mention flexible sex! It also has the aphrodisiac spices fennel, nutmeg and garlic.

Prep Time	Cook Time
20 min	20 min

Course	Lunch/Dinner
Serves	4-6

Ingredients

2 large potatoes
1 head kale
32 oz low sodium broth
1 half-gallon carton of coconut milk
1 large handful of fresh chopped parsley
1 Tbsp olive oil
1 chopped onion
2 Tbsp fennel seeds
3/4 tsp nutmeg
1 tsp black pepper
Salt to taste (less is better for great sex)

Instructions

1. Heat olive oil in a large pot. Add onion, fennel and nutmeg and cook until onion is translucent and spices are aromatic.
2. Add other ingredients, minus coconut milk, bringing to a boil and simmering until potatoes are cooked through.
3. Add coconut milk and heat through.
4. Serve with a salad of your choice.

Spiced Butternut Squash Soup

Creamy sex-healthy butternut squash soup made with very little fat for better genital blood flow. Squash is a great source of potassium, which has an immediate benefit to vascular function. Plus this soup is loaded with natural aphrodisiacs such as nutmeg and garlic, the better for your load.

Prep Time	Cook Time
20 min	20 min
Course	Lunch/Dinner
Serves	6

Ingredients

1 large butternut squash
2 Tbsp butter or coconut cream
1 medium onion, sliced
3 cloves garlic, minced
2 tsp cinnamon (or more to taste)
1 tsp cardamom (or more to taste)
1/8 tsp nutmeg
1 quart low-sodium vegetable broth
4 Tbsp pure maple syrup
Salt to taste (less is better for great sex)

Instructions

1. Preheat oven to 400°F. Cut butternut squash in half lengthwise and scoop out seeds. Place both halves flesh-side down on a parchment paper-lined baking sheet. Bake for about an hour, until tender.
2. While squash cools, melt 2 tablespoons of butter or coconut cream in a large pot over medium heat. Once melted, add in onion and cook until soft and translucent, about 8 minutes.
3. Next add in garlic, cinnamon, cardamom and nutmeg. Cook 1-2 minutes until fragrant.
4. Pour in vegetable broth.

5. Scoop out flesh from roasted squash and add it to your pot. Cook for 5-10 minutes to meld flavors then transfer to a high-powered blender and blend until smooth or use an immersion blender in the pot.

6. With the heat off, add in maple syrup, salt and any additional spices to taste.

7. Top with whatever you like! You can drizzle it with coconut milk, cardamom, cinnamon, roasted seeds, hot sauce and red pepper flakes for a little kick!

Recipe from Emily Daniels at Wholesome Hedonista. For full video, visit: https://www.instagram.com/p/B-piis-pkwf/

My Sunday Sauce

This sauce tastes amazing and is loaded with sex-healthy, antioxidant-rich vegetables with a few aphrodisiac spices thrown in as well. I used to make this sauce with loads of meat, but I found that it really isn't necessary. The fennel, nutmeg, chile peppers and parsley give it a rich, Italian sausage flavor without the excessive fat, to keep you light and agile in bed.

Prep Time	Cook Time
30 min	20 min (3 hours if fresh tomatoes)
Course	Dinner
Serves	4

Ingredients

6 huge tomatoes, homegrown and in season is best. You can also use 2 32oz cans of tomato sauce if you prefer
8 oz sliced fresh mushrooms. I like to use plain white, oyster and lion's mane
1 cup chopped kale
1 onion
1/4 cup fennel seeds
3/4 tsp nutmeg
1/2 tsp ground nutmeg
2 jalapeños, or chiles finely diced, or more if you like it spicy
2 cloves garlic
A handful of chopped fresh parsley
1/4 cup fresh basil chopped
1 tsp fresh chopped oregano
Salt and pepper to taste (less salt is better for great sex)
A drizzle of olive oil (less is better for great sex)

Instructions

1. Slice tomatoes and boil down until proper sauce consistency. Or use canned sauce.
2. Add chopped kale and simmer.
3. In a non-stick skillet, heat olive oil and add fennel, nutmeg and garlic. Cook for one minute, until fragrant. Add onions and cook until translucent. Add to the pot.
4. Add remaining ingredients and simmer for 15 minutes (longer if you are using fresh tomatoes).
5. Serve over pasta. I prefer brown rice pasta.

The Best Guacamole and Salsa Ever!

You can use the base to make either salsa, guacamole or both! This delicious sex snack is loaded with antioxidants, vitamin C, E and, for the guac, PUFAs.

Prep Time	Cook Time
20 min	0

Course	Appetizer/Snack
Serves	6

Ingredients

Base

3 cloves garlic
1 bunch scallions
2 jalapeños
2 limes, juiced
1 bunch cilantro
A pinch of salt or to taste

For Guacamole

Add 2 avocados

Or for Salsa

Add 2 tomatoes
1/2 tsp cumin
1 Tbsp tomato paste
1 tsp maple syrup or honey

Instructions

1. Mix all of the base ingredients in a food processor until finely chopped.
2. For guacamole, add 2 avocados and blend in the food processor until creamy.
3. For Salsa, omit avocado and add tomatoes, cumin, tomato paste and maple syrup. Pulse until coarsely chopped.
4. Serve with tortilla chips. Or use it to top a burrito bowl or beans and rice.

Pink Fluffy Nice Cream

This amazing pink fluffy nice cream is made completely from fruit. High in potassium and antioxidants, it luxuriates blood vessels and nerves leading to and from the genitals for a sweet tooth and a sweet night of passion.

Prep Time	Cook Time
20 min	0
Course	Dessert
Serves	3-4

Ingredients

5 frozen, sliced bananas

1/2 cup fresh or frozen pink pitaya (dragon fruit) (You can use raspberries or blueberries instead)

A splash of almond milk or water (only if needed for consistency)

Instructions

1. Blend in a high-powered blender until creamy.
2. Add toppings of your choice such as slivered almonds or toasted coconut.
3. If you'd like to add more color, add some blue spirulina.

Recipe from Emily Daniels at Wholesome Hedonista. For full video, visit: https://www.instagram.com/p/B7oKBQBpkFI/

Sex Juice

This drink is appropriately named as it gets the juices flowing with nitrate-rich beets, which boost nitric oxide for great blood flow and great sex. In addition, aphrodisiac ginger and chiles deliciously spice things up.

Prep Time	Cook Time
5 min	0

Course	Breakfast/Snack
Serves	1

Ingredients

A bunch of fresh beets (pomegranates or fennel bulb are also good, if you don't like beets)
1 spicy pepper of your choice, such as poblano or jalapeño
Thumb of ginger

Instructions

1. Juice all ingredients and enjoy! If you don't like beets, you can substitute with fennel bulb or pomegranates, and feel free to add a dash of ground cloves, saffron or nutmeg.

Iced Chaga Chai Latte

Did you know that chaga has more antioxidants per gram than açaí, pomegranates and blueberries combined? And chaga was used in WWII as a coffee substitute because it has a delicate vanilla flavor. This delicious iced drink combines mushrooms, which speed nerve conduction to and from genitals, with aphrodisiac spices such as fennel and nutmeg. Get your juices flowing!

Prep Time	Cook Time
40 min	20 min
Course	Drink
Serves	2

Ingredients

4-5 large chaga chunks
2 cups water
2 cups almond milk
A pinch of cardamom
A pinch of cinnamon
A pinch of nutmeg
A pinch of fennel or ginger
1/4 tsp vanilla
2 -3 Tbsp honey or maple syrup
Ice (2 glasses filled)

Instructions

1. Gently boil chaga chunks until the water is a deep brown color, like espresso, about 25 minutes. The chaga chunks can then be dried and reused. With each use it takes longer to boil. Or you can use more chunks to make a big pot and store it in the fridge.
2. Add spices and honey. Stir.
3. Pour over ice, filling 1/3 of a glass. Add almond milk to fill to the top.

4. Enjoy this delicious treat, which you can adjust to your preference of spiciness and sweetness.

Recipe from Emily Daniels at Wholesome Hedonista. For full video, visit: https://www.instagram.com/p/B9U8cv-JVVL/

Mangonada

This traditional Mexican drink contains mango, abundant in antioxidants and potassium. This makes for penile and clitoral arterial and nerve health and free-flowing sex. Mangonada is cool, refreshing, sweet, smokey and a little spicy! Enjoy this on a hot day or to spice up (literally) your morning smoothie ritual. It's naturally sweetened by all the delicious fruit and has virtually no fat!

Prep Time	Cook Time
10 min	0
Course	Drink
Serves	2

Ingredients

Mango Smoothie Base

4 cups fresh or frozen mango chunks
2 cups orange juice, adjust for consistency
Fresh lime juice

Chamoy Sauce

1/2 cup dried apricot
1/2 small fresh apricot
1/2 dried ancho chile
1 Tbsp maple syrup
4 tsp chile powder
1 lime, juiced
3/4 cup water
1/8 tsp (or less) salt

Instructions

1. Blend mango smoothie ingredients in a blender until smooth.

2. To make the chamoy sauce, soak apricot and dried chile in water for about 10 minutes to ease blending.

3. Blend all chamoy sauce ingredients together until smooth. You may have to add more liquid.

4. Coat the rim of a glass with lime juice, then dip in chili powder for a coated rim.

5. Drizzle the inner sides of the glass with the chamoy sauce, then pour in mango smoothie.

6. Drizzle a bit of chamoy sauce over the top and enjoy! This drink is traditionally served with a tamarind straw, which you can find at a Mexican grocery or make your own using the online recipe, but that is completely optional.

Recipe from Emily Daniels at Wholesome Hedonista. For video, visit: https://www.instagram.com/p/B4xcl2UlEEI/

BONUS: A FEW TIPS TO GIVE YOU SOME GAME IN THE BEDROOM

Here is a tale of two orgasms.

Steven's wife controlled sex in the relationship. It was understood that he needed it, and she rationed it out like gold stars if he behaved himself. When he was single, he loved getting head from lovers for no special reason at all, especially the ones who really seemed to *like* it.

Here with his wife, though, "like" was more like grin and bear it. He was afraid to communicate his sexual desires to her because she always seemed to disapprove. Not helping matters was the fact that she openly admitted she thought that semen was disgusting, and when he would ejaculate, she would act annoyed and say, "Ewww," cleaning it up immediately. He loved his wife, but felt very dissatisfied sexually.

Rita, on the other hand, eagerly gave her partner head almost every time they were intimate, yet he never got the message, and only went down on her on special occasions. When he did perform oral sex on her, it wasn't exactly pleasurable. He didn't seem to like the way female genitals smelled and tasted, leaving her self-conscious throughout the entire ordeal.

As he didn't focus on clitoral stimulation, she needed her vibrator to orgasm, and he complained that the noise was a turn-off. As a result, she rarely had an orgasm with her partner. She loved him, but her feelings were souring as she realized he was indifferent to her needs.

Steven and Rita's stories illustrate something very important: We all want our partner to adore us, and what better way than to taste the most intimate part of their body. So go down on each other. Do it often, do it freely. Do it enthusiastically. Do it maniacally. Do it like there is no tomorrow. Do it for each other. Do it for your country.

Go Down to Get Up (And Get Off)

In all seriousness, there is no way around this fact: In order to call ourselves good lovers, we must know how to give good head. Because when our partner does this for us, it makes us feel nurtured and it makes us feel special. And best of all, feeling adored helps lower our inhibition so we can relax, enjoy and fully participate in sex. And for this, we are immensely grateful to our partners and closer to boot.

It is truly staggering how many relationships are one-sided in this respect, with one partner doing the heavy lifting and the other sitting back and enjoying the ride. Though between heterosexual couples, the sex act typically begins and ends with male orgasm, more likely to leave women in the lurch, we've discussed that the one-sidedness can come from either side in the relationship, in relationships of any orientation.

But we are duty bound as good lovers to challenge that selfish side, the part in all of us who greedily wants all of the pleasure for ourselves. Those of us uninterested in anything but our own pleasure are better suited to the services of a sex worker, who will at least be handsomely compensated for tending only to us with no expectation of return pleasure.

For those of us interested in maintaining partnerships which are less transactional, taking the time to learn how to go down on your partner is a fundamental act of kindness. It is you giving to your partner, taking care of their needs. And, as is true of all acts of kindness, the rewards are so much sweeter when we give than when we receive.

I understand that for many of us, we *are* invested in our partner's pleasure, but hit obstacles along the way. Through lack of experience or lack of education, some of us don't know our partners butt from a hole in the wall.

People often complain that their partner doesn't know what the hell they're doing down there. But, as gently as I can put this, that is pure laziness. Bringing pleasure to ones partner is usually just a matter of caring enough to learn and not letting our ego get in the way of that learning.

Learning how to please a female body can be especially challenging, and loads of partners don't make the effort, or they place the responsibility on her, but some males can be tricky too. Given the plethora of information that abounds online about how to do this, we have little in the way of excuses.

Bringing new techniques to the bedroom from our own research and reading is great because it creates an opportunity to communicate with our partner and get crucial feedback. Simple questions like, "Does this feel good?" and "What would feel better?" are powerful tools toward having mutually satisfying sex.

Fortunately, with a bit of practice, there is enough information here to please even the most discerning penises and vulvas.

Giving the Penis a Head Start

The penis seems like a pretty straightforward situation, a series of unruly ups and downs, to be sure, but relatively easy to master if you approach it right. Put simply, the penis needs to be worshipped.

To that end, enthusiasm is more than half the battle here. Those who give head best are generally ones who enjoy doing it. For anyone who says, "Well, I don't like doing it, so I'll never be good," remember that such perspectives all but seal your fate. You *do* have a choice as to how you view oral sex, just as you have a choice about how you view other things that might be unfamiliar to you.

And though I've never met your partner, I know this: He would most likely love it if you gave head like the only thing you want in that moment is his dick in your mouth. It's a big turn on. So if it helps, try reminding yourself of that as a mantra before you begin. After all, pleasing your partner is the point. Getting in the mindset that you hold the key to his ultimate pleasure can feel empowering and exciting.

It's true that some men are apprehensive about getting head because they worry that their partner won't like the way that they taste or smell, their hairiness or their size. They also worry that if they orgasm from oral, they won't be able to pleasure you with penetration. Nobody wants to disappoint.

But enthusiasm on your part comes right back into play here. The worst possible feeling is getting head from someone who is not-so-patiently waiting for you to come so they can be done with it. When you give head, leave other acts off the table. This is an end to itself. Forget the rest, clear your mind and focus on one thing and one thing only.

Be sure to cultivate the pleasure you feel in tasting your partner and don't be afraid to vocalize it. Your pleasure is his pleasure, and it eases any worries he has about whether or not you are happy with his junk.

Of note, gay male couples tend to more easily understand the importance of loving their partner's penis, as owners of penises themselves. But hetero women, on the other hand, often inadvertently make their man feel bad about his. Don't. Men are just as inundated with genital insecurity. As they tend to watch more porn than women, they're misled to believe that what women want is a long dong. They've also ignored that for every dozen or so dicks a woman may have encountered, men are operating off the cumulative image of hundreds of monster dicks to compare with their normal-sized one.

The Smeller's the Feller

A note about male odor. Even when someone has great hygiene, and washes just prior to sex, the penis and testicles have a natural male odor. Your partner hopes you like his. Just as it enhances the female sexual experience to have a partner who likes your vulva, and its natural fragrance, this is also very important to men.

When their partner genuinely likes the look, feel, smell and taste of their penis, it can provide a variety of sexual enhancements. It can increase his sexual arousal, boost his confidence, and also ease some of the anxiety and insecurities that are normal to feel during sex. It's important to develop an appreciation for the penis, and also to learn about the anatomy of it.

How to Give Great Head

Start slow. Give a preview of what's to come. Touch and caress him over his pants or underwear. When he is naked, take the time to admire the sight of him. Kiss his chest, abdomen, thighs. Rub your face gently against his penis, or brush your lips against his inguinal area and give a little tongue if you like. Take your time and let yours and his arousal build naturally. Anticipation adds to the excitement of getting head.

Kiss the head of his penis and slowly lick the frenulum on the underside. This part of a penis is loaded with nerves, so it is a particularly pleasurable spot.

The most common way to give head is to gently suck and lick the head of the penis and part of the shaft while stroking the rest of the shaft with your hand. This technique works quite well. You can stroke up and down, or make an O with your hand and gently rotate back and forth while taking his penis in and out of your mouth. So, basically, if you can pat your head and rub your belly at the same time, you can give good head.

To enhance pleasure, or go hands-free, you can stimulate the head, frenulum and shaft simultaneously using just your mouth. With the penis inside the back of the mouth, gently squeeze the head of his penis between the base of the tongue and the roof of your mouth, toward or including the soft palette, as your lips apply pressure to the shaft of the penis. Gently take the penis in and out of the mouth while using your tongue to massage his frenulum and shaft. Giving head this way allows optimal stimulation of the head and frenulum, while stroking his shaft with your lips. This can be intensely pleasurable for him. But be mindful that he may come very quickly this way.

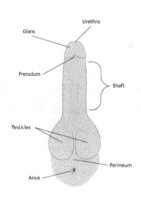

Underside View of the Male Genitals

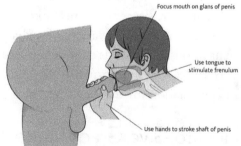

Focus Stimulation on Glans of Penis

Hot Tips

- Lots of guys like visual stimulation. It turns them on to see your body and also to watch as their penis goes in and out of your mouth. Many also like it when you maintain eye contact while giving them head.

- Remember that the glans is the most sensitive part of the penis. Lighter pressure is applied here. Heavier pressure on the shaft. Men generally prefer though, that you maintain some kind of suction or contact with the glans throughout.

- Your tongue is a very important part of giving good head. Remember that your tongue has both a tip for zeroing in on a particular spot and a broad flat center. Each can add pleasure. You can use it to massage his penis while taking it in and out of your mouth. You can also use it to flick the frenulum or lick the sides of his head and shaft.

- Pay attention to the response you're getting from him to guide you in how much pressure you use. If you need help, don't be afraid to ask.

- Gently tug, caress, lick or suck his balls if he enjoys that. It is also quite pleasurable to lick the perineum, or area between the anus and scrotum. Or caress the base of the penis.

- Some guys like it when you periodically move from his penis to his testicles, and especially his perineum, with your mouth and tongue. Others prefer that, once you get to the good part, you stay right there.

- Many guys like it when you massage the perineum or insert a finger into the anus while giving head. This stimulates the male G-spot, or prostate. You may want to ask first.

- Faster isn't necessarily better. Slow and sensual is also good. Don't be impatient. If it's taking longer than you think, it doesn't mean that you aren't doing it right.

- For those of you with a stronger gag reflex, simply take it slow. The more time you spend with his penis in the back of your throat, breathing normally, the more relaxed you will become and the less-pronounced the gag reflex will be. You can also practice desensitization when brushing your teeth. If you routinely brush the back of your tongue, your gag reflex will lessen. If taking him into your mouth deeply just isn't working for you, you can focus on using your hands more to stroke his shaft and moving over the glans while only the topmost part of the penis is in the mouth.

- Avoid scraping his penis with your teeth. This can cause pain and injury.
- If the penis has foreskin, this can be a site of pleasure. It feels good to stimulate it with your mouth and tongue.
- If you get fatigued, you can switch to using your hand to glide up and down over the shaft and glans of the penis. You can also lick their glans, especially the frenulum, while stimulating him manually, which gives your jaw a rest but allows him to feel your tongue. It's kind of like giving a good hand job with some mouth and tongue.
- Many males say that it's a big turn-on when their partner swallows their semen. It's certainly not essential though. Some also enjoy coming on their partner's face or other parts of the body.
- The most common complaint when receiving head is pain: when their partner sucks too hard like a vacuum cleaner, squeezes the testicles too hard or any use of teeth.

That Big O: The Elusive Female Orgasm

As sought-after as the orgasm is for everyone, consider that heterosexual women have the fewest of all.[413] This is unfortunate but easily explained: Males can typically climax with penetrative sex, a hand job or a blow job, meaning the in and out or up and down will usually get the job done.

Females, on the other hand, need clitoral stimulation and/or penetrative action. Yes, some women can orgasm from sex alone, and research suggests this is related to the distance between the clitoris and vaginal opening (more on this in a moment). Lesbians tend to become more proficient at getting women off, with the added knowledge of similar working parts.

But before you get out a measuring stick, you should just take any woman's word for it: Whatever she needs is whatever it takes.

The most important thing you can take away from this is a corrective to a longstanding myth or misunderstanding that women somehow don't care about whether they get off. That they don't need to as much as men do.

The reality is that they've had to get used to less getting off, though it certainly needn't be this way. That myth is perpetuated in many ways, and sometimes by women themselves (we'll get to that in a moment). But even recently, I came across an article in a men's magazine explaining to women that men are very insecure about being able to give a woman an orgasm. And men should know, the author continued, that sex is the main attraction for women, not orgasm.

His advice? That women should reassure their partners, explaining that, "Simply telling them [the guy] that your goal is not a big orgasm will lead to a better time for everyone involved." I wondered if "everyone" included her.

We all can sympathize that dating and sex can be terrifying and brings out our deepest insecurities and feelings of inadequacy. Having said this, I assure you that this guy is out of line. Women want orgasms. They want big orgasms. They want lots of orgasms.

The fact is, that, if we are using the male standard as our measuring stick, then women are a little bit trickier to please than men. But that doesn't make getting them off a complex algorithm, nor does it mean it's impossible or even difficult.

It just means you have to actually figure out what she responds to. And that means you have to actually make an effort. Effort is a key word here! Men seemingly climax with little or no effort, so we've concluded that any effort is difficult. It isn't! It's just effort.

Most women will also be quite patient with you if you just try to do this—after all, like you, they want to get off. If your female partner does not climax, this may not have anything to do with you or what you are doing. But it might.

I'll Have What She's Having

That said, we have to address the fake orgasm. Like it or not, many, many women fake orgasms. (Some men have been known to, as well!) Usually, men respond to this with disbelief. Why would anyone fake one of the greatest experiences on earth!?! Well, it's because of what happens when they don't. (What happens is nothing, meaning no orgasm, or worse, male disappointment, frustration or even anger.)

In order to understand why women fake it, you have to understand about the female sexual experience from their perspective. Once they've realized that climax won't be coming, they feel it's the only expected way to conclude sex.

It is done with other good intentions. They want their partner to feel competent, to feel the experience of having satisfied their desires. They don't want to hurt their partner's feelings. I've heard women say, "Well, it's never going to happen, so why make him feel bad?"

I know that we all deal with our insecurities, and I wouldn't want to make anyone feel bad either. But if someone wants the experience of pleasing a woman without taking the time to educate themselves about the female anatomy and how to optimally stimulate it, then they haven't earned it.

To be clear, some women feel that they just can't orgasm with a partner. That it takes too long and that they are just happy (read: resigned to) sharing the intimacy without the big finish for them. While this may be a valid point for a smaller percentage of women, for most it is simply that they and their partners may not have adequate knowledge. According to science, most women (at least 80%) can and do orgasm with their partners.

While men take an average of six minutes to achieve orgasm, women take much longer. One study[414] found that *after* a female is intensely aroused, she takes an average of fourteen minutes to climax when with a partner, and many women take significantly longer. While masturbating, on the other hand, it took women an average of eight minutes.

What this means is that taking the time to build a woman's arousal and subsequent climax could easily take thirty minutes to an hour. Of course there is great variation for individuals. And the more you learn about her body, and the more turned on she is, the more relaxed she feels and the faster this will go. But fast isn't necessarily the goal here. Building to pleasure is a valid, intrinsically good outcome when it comes to sex—quickies are great, too, but leisurely lovemaking has many merits.

If a woman tells you not to worry about her orgasm, that she is enjoying herself with just the intimacy, consider that there are two possibilities and the second is the much more likely one.

Reason One: For physiological or psychological reasons she simply can't orgasm (see the section on Female Orgasmic Disorder, FOD).

Reason Two: Her experience with you and other partners has shown her that they don't know how to touch her in a way that is pleasurable and leads to orgasm.

The first scenario needs a bit more investigation, but for many women, it's the second scenario, and that's one you can address right there at home.

In addition to her being conditioned to expect not to get off from others, or with you, she's likely to have added some logic as to why.

She likely thinks you couldn't possibly be interested in sitting there for forty-five minutes just for her pleasure, just to figure it out. Though we have made a lot of progress, women have been taught that their wants and needs are not as important as their partner's. That expecting or demanding pleasure entirely for themselves is selfish.

Consider, also, that most women have extensive experience with partners who make it obvious that they don't have the time for her pleasure, only theirs. They express frustration, make jokes about sore jaws or outright complain. Worse, some men will accuse those women of not wanting them or even being unfaithful.

And finally, she may simply imagine those partners don't know how to properly stimulate a woman sexually and not know how to even address this or where to begin.

Porn: Titillating, Not Always Telling

Porn, while it might be good for getting your juices flowing, or introducing you to new positions or sexual acrobatics, is not necessarily going to help here. Though it has increasingly begun to show more realistic depictions of female pleasure, you still have to look for that, and most of it relies on lazy theatrics that suggest women orgasm effortlessly and with nothing but the sight of a penis.

And still, there's this woman in front of you, who may or may not respond to any of those things. Again, you'll need to inquire about this woman's needs and particular preferences. In fact, many women themselves do not realize that they are capable of orgasm with a partner and do not even know specific techniques to advise their partner.

Knowing how to please a woman involves an extensive education, not just a quick browse of the internet. It means you have a nice toolbox of tricks to test on *each* partner individually. You include your fingers (vaginally or anally); you are licking the clit and not the part next to it. You know the difference between the outer hood of the clit versus the inner most-sensitive part, and that each person likes different pressure and speed.

Guys want to give their partner an orgasm and feel inadequate if they don't, but this is true even for the suckiest of lovers. What's hard for women to understand is this: If guys are so insecure about giving a woman an orgasm, why do so few of them ever take the time to learn?

When I think back on my own experience, I realize that many of my boyfriends had this same insecurity, and I see that I handled it like most women do, by assuring them that I was very happy with their sexual performance.

And I thought this because I didn't know any better. I didn't realize that sex could be way more pleasurable if my partner had a stronger skill set. What I should have done was asked them if they could please pick up a book on the subject, or better yet, a couple books, and talk to a few lesbians who could share some tips. I also should've been able to better articulate what I might like better.

These men were not uniquely selfish or indifferent. Their efforts demonstrated that they *wanted* to be good lovers but they hadn't done the leg work. These are guys who used very few of the techniques that actually work on women. The ones we will talk about.

A good lover will master a varied approach to pleasure so that they can give their partner the most and best orgasms. And if she simply does not orgasm, they will at least optimize her pleasure. And, as always, they'll continue to explore options, fueled by the desire to unlock this woman's pleasure and enhance their experience mutually.

The Dick is Not a Magic Wand

Remember I mentioned that some women can orgasm from intercourse alone? According to one large study,[415] that's only about 18% of women. Most women, about 70%, need clitoral stimulation in order to get the job done.[416]

So you can search the ends of the earth until you find that woman (yardstick in hand), but you'll never be quite sure she isn't just faking unless you discuss her specific needs and preferences.

The point here: Don't feel insulted if your dick alone cannot finish the job. There is a reason for this. In the medical community it's called CUMD—and, no, it's not the past tense of cum. It actually stands for Clitoral Urethral Meatus Distance. What this means is that some women have a much shorter distance between the vagina and clitoris, and for this reason, their clitoris can be stimulated during intercourse by the motion of sex itself, the pressure of your body against her, and the way you position yourself within her.

Hey, I'm sure most women would be thrilled to have this situation, but unfortunately this accounts for only about 25%[417] of women. For the rest of us, our clitoris is just too far away to be stimulated, so the poor thing gets left out in the traditional wham-bam.

But the more orgasms she has, the better in touch with her body she is, and the more likely she is to help you get her there together. According to research,[418] women who do have more orgasms have a few things in common. These women receive more oral sex, longer sex, they are more satisfied in their relationships, and they aren't afraid to ask for what they want in bed. These women also seem to have a more positive, playful attitude toward their partners and toward sex in general. They are more likely to praise their partner for something they did sexually or to send them a note later in the day to tease them about something sexual. They are more open to trying new positions and to talking dirty.

Physiology of Female Orgasm

The physiology of the female orgasm is not fully understood, but there are certain things that we do know:
1. Women become aroused when either we think about something sexual or there is physical stimulation to the breasts, clitoris, vagina or other erogenous zones.
2. The clitoris is the most densely innervated part of the female human body. Blood engorges the clitoris just as it does the penis.
3. Stimulation of the clitoris stimulates nerve endings, which send signals to the brain.
4. The brain processes these signals, translating them to sexual pleasure which culminates in a flood of dopamine and intense pleasure.

Female Orgasmic Disorder

Low libido is the most common female sexual complaint. The second most common sexual issue for women is female orgasmic disorder (FOD). FOD is a medical condition characterized by inability or difficulty achieving orgasm despite adequate stimulation of the genitals. A total of 40% of women report difficulty achieving orgasm and 20% report complete inability to achieve it.

Causes can include underlying medical conditions such as obesity, diabetes and cardiovascular disease. There are emotional and psychological reasons too, such as interpersonal and relationship issues, self-esteem and/ or body issues.

An international collaboration of urology and sexual medicine experts assembled the Disorders of Orgasm in Women Committee[419] to review evidence-based effective treatment for women for this issue. But extensive review of available medical literature revealed that there are no *drugs* currently available that are more effective than placebo in treating FOD. Viagra has demonstrated sexual benefits to women in research but is only approved by the FDA for use with men.

However, there are effective treatments of another sort that were identified by this committee. Those included cognitive-behavioral therapy, where a therapist helps to change thought processes associated with sex, reduce anxiety and improve communication with their partner.

They may also teach the person to embrace the sensory pleasures, and to use Kegel exercises. Additionally, sufferers may be given behavioral exercises to perform at home, such as directed masturbation to establish comfort with looking at and touching oneself. Kegel exercises strengthen the pelvic floor and increase blood flow to the genitals, which has been shown to improve sexual satisfaction and orgasmic function.[420]

There are both physiological and psycho-social factors that may contribute to FOD, including history of sexual abuse, anxiety, depression, feeling rejection during intercourse and poor communication with one's partner.

Therein lies the rub for women. Sometimes we make the issue of orgasm overly complex. For many women, all they've really needed is a willing partner, eager to help them sort out their particular combination.

Thus, it's not surprising that masturbation was a technique used effectively in many studies! Basically, women who masturbate know their bodies well enough to instruct their partners how to please them. Of course, women who don't feel sexual gratification from masturbation have less incentive to do so. However, research has shown that sexual activity leads to short-term increases in testosterone, which can affect sexual desire and gratification.

But culturally, we don't celebrate, encourage or at least expect and accept female masturbation the way we do in teenage boys and men. The result is fewer women are in touch with their bodies' central pleasure spots. And often, lifetimes of unfulfilling sexual experiences.

That wouldn't make anyone feel too confident about getting off. And anxiety has been shown in research to be a major obstacle to achieving orgasm. Sometimes it is her very concerns over difficulty achieving orgasm that lead to her anxiety, which makes it harder to orgasm, which increases anxiety.

I had a patient in my practice whose boyfriend always made her feel like she was defective because he could come on command and it took her substantially longer. That, in a nutshell, is the entire problem.

The first part of this book extensively discusses helping the female body to have a better physiological sexual response through diet. The strategies there can make a huge difference in clitoral sensitivity and ability to orgasm. But none of them will result in climax without addressing these simple distinctions in how women get off, and it is your job as a partner to discover the solution.

The Pampered Pussy

The female sexual experience is unique in that orgasm is a gift that is not guaranteed. She and her partner must work for it, being equally invested in her pleasure, just as much as they are in their own pleasure.

You should know that many women, too, worry about certain things when you go down on them. What if you don't like her vagina? What if you think it smells bad? Don't like the taste? That's in addition to any insecurities she may have about her body and being naked in front of you.

A simple truth: A woman is not likely to climax if she is feeling self-conscious. That's where you come in. You can either make her feel defective or you can make her feel like a goddess, which will relax her nerves, increase pleasure and ease orgasm.

There are still some people who feel that it is perfectly ok to receive oral sex and not reciprocate. It is *sometimes*, just as it's ok to solely focus on your partner's needs occasionally.

But in general we should aim to give at least as much as we receive. This is particularly important for guys, who have a reputation for falling short here. Believe me, it is *not* just as gratifying for her to give head to a partner who does not make the same effort. When we just think about our own needs, we end up with partners who feel unfulfilled.

A Rating System for Oral Sex

Statistically, it's impossible to know how many guys out there are great at going down. There is certainly a wide variation in how proficient men are in giving oral sex to a woman.

Due to this ambiguity, I've devised my personal rating system for oral sex. Keep in mind, my experience is limited to men, but also keep in mind that it's usually straight males who need the most work in this area. Female pussy eaters tend to be more skilled at it, likely because they themselves know how different techniques feel.

Cunninlingus Rubric: How to Ace Your Orals		
Grade	Criteria	Percent of males* falling into this category
A+	The tongue consistently produces strong pleasure on point and at appropriate (to her) pressure. Can deliver an orgasm better than she can herself. Uses both the flat surface of the tongue as well as the tip. Is skilled at using adjunctive techniques such as vaginal or anal fingering and nipple stimulation, depending on her preference. Communicates and is responsive to cues from her. Those who score A+ are exceptionally invested in their partner's pleasure, and have usually put considerable effort into learning about a wide variety of strategies for pleasing her.	Less than 5%

B	Usually the tongue is stimulating appropriately to produce at least some pleasure. Uses adjunctive techniques such as vaginal or anal fingering or nipple stimulation. With some time and patience, orgasm is possible. People scoring in the B range need to remember to reinvent their technique with each new partner. Being better than 80% of other lovers seems pretty good, but with some initiative, you could move into A range. Even though your last girlriend liked it, you need to explore what this girl likes.	15%
C	Sometimes on point and pleasurable, but often misses the mark. Pressure is often too light to produce pleasure, or too hard as to be over-stimulating. May not use adjunctive techniques such as fingering. These are people who looked up how to give head once online, too cues from porn, or asked a buddy, and feel that they now have a full toolbox.	35%
D	Occasionally on point and pleasurable. She's noticing cracks in the ceiling because that is more interesting than what's going on down there. May be thinking of what she needs from the grocery store, while hoping her grunts are convincing. After all, its awfully nice of him to do that for her, so she wants him to know how wonderful he is.	25%
F	Very little ability to produce pleasure. May have indicated an aversion to the pussy, or its taste, smell etc. These are usually people who dislike performing oral sex, or sex in general, or are only concerned about their own pleasure.	20%

* Female pussy-eaters tend to be much more proficient than indicated by these percentages.

The biggest complaints that women have about their partner's techniques are as follows:

- When their partner uses the wrong pressure. Too little brings no pleasure at all. Too much can be unpleasant and overstimulating. Just communicate. The more you learn about your partner, the better you can pleasure her.

- Missing the mark. *Most* men have a pattern like this: If the clit were a bullseye, every lick oscillates between hitting and missing the mark, like repeatedly hitting a piñata blindfolded.

Can you imagine how difficult it would be to orgasm under those circumstances? The tutorial below will train you how to consistently be on point.

Real-Life Mr. Pussy

Every now and then, someone comes along who is a pussy-eating superstar. This is the one we *wish* it could have worked out with because then we would have gotten that special attention for years to come.

There was a guy I dated who I refer to fondly as a real-life Mr. Pussy. The reason was simple: He was the rare breed that could deliver an orgasm better than I could myself. He loved doing it, that much was clear. And as a result of this magical combination of enthusiasm and skill, he was not just a little better, he was leagues better.

Lest you think he is lucky, or has something you don't, let's take a look at what made him this way. Such superstars of oral have a few things in common.

They Care Enough to Learn

As noted above extensively, men who excel at oral don't just take their tips from porn. It's not just from reading primers on the internet. They care enough to ask their partners what they like, but not as if it were a formal interview. They also pay attention to what their partner's respond to and don't. They understand female anatomy but try lots of different techniques, understanding that not one move fits all.

If you want to make your partner happy, you must try lots of different things while communicating with your partner, to see what she likes. And you must get your information from a variety of sources. After spending a whole lot of time doing this, you will become *very* good at it. When you are with a woman for the first time, she will want more of what you're bringing.

They Love the Yoni

Men who really shine at giving head not only *like* the female genitalia, they love it. The sight, smell and taste of it turns them on.

Hopefully your partner will be considerate and freshen up for you beforehand, but even so, genitals, both male and female, have a natural biological aroma and taste. I am aware that this may be an acquired taste. But nobody ever liked gorgonzola or a fine aged wine the first time they tried it. They built up positive feelings associated with that taste and smell until they began to relish it. Your partner hopes you like her taste and smell.

One of the hottest things is dating someone who loves your pussy. A friend told me how, before he would go down on her, her boyfriend liked to get his face very close to her yoni with the lights on and touch himself. He loved seeing, touching and tasting hers. That was a big turn-on for her.

Conversely, many women recount experiences with partners who don't like their genitals. It's obvious because they don't spend too much time down there experiencing it up close and personal. They act squeamish about touching and tasting them.

This can definitely spoil her arousal. Yet many of these partners wanted to feel like competent lovers. But a partner who doesn't like our genitals can make us feel unattractive and uncared for. That's why anyone who wants to please a woman should cultivate their appreciation for the pussy.

People who achieve Oral God status also *enjoy* giving head. If you are bored, and counting down the minutes, believe me, your partner will know it. She won't be able to relax and enjoy herself knowing that you're not into it. Conversely, someone who is just loving having their face between your legs is really hot!

They Adjust According to Their Partner's Preferences

Don't make oral about you or your ego. It's quite counterproductive to the entire point here, which is adoring your partner. Oral is about sharing intimacy and appreciating each other's bodies. It's your time to give to her, and hopefully you will enjoy that just as much as receiving pleasure.

Don't just accept or endure feedback. *Invite* feedback. Ask your partner,

"Do you like this better or this?" And if she does speak up, encourage her. It may have been hard for her to say because she didn't want to hurt your feelings.

Don't let your pride get in the way of becoming an expert pussy-eater. If you make it uncomfortable for her to guide you, you will not grow as quickly as a lover. Also, once we learn something, we tend to become know-it-alls. This woman is different from the last one, so you don't yet know about her. Extra hint: Don't ever mention when she doesn't like something that it went over like gangbusters with another woman.

A Lesbian's Guide to Eating Pussy

Males and females are different, and while some people can get off any which way the wind blows, she can't. Cultivating the art of cunnilingus requires time and patience. Are you game? If you put your mind to it, you can be the lover that every woman remembers. The one who cared about her pleasure enough to savor it. Relish it. Bathe in it.

I thought I knew what good head was. There were guys who did it well, and guys who didn't. One day though, my lesbian friend gave me a lesson, and I was astounded at what she said. Of course, I thought, who better to mentor on the subject than someone who both has her pussy and eats it too. In her step-by-step instructions, she described things that no one had ever done for me, which I then communicated to my partner.

As a result of my dear friend, oral sex was a completely different experience, well worth taking the time to learn.

Advanced Pussy Eating

The tutorial below is based on the expertise of the aforementioned, highly accomplished pussy-eaters.

- Have her lie on her back. For yours and her comfort, you can place a pillow below her bottom. You won't have to crook your neck as much. It is quite comfortable to kneel on the floor while she lies on the bed, possibly with her legs on your shoulders. If you both don't mind something a little different, you can also have her lie on the kitchen table while you sit in a chair in front of her.

- Start slow. There's more to a pussy than the clit, so don't go straight for it. Give a preview of what's to come. Touch and caress her body, her legs, her breasts. Feel her pussy over the outside of her underwear. When she is naked, take the time to relish the sight of her. Rub your face gently against her pubis or brush your lips against her inguinal area and give a little tongue if you like. Take your time and let yours and her arousal build naturally. Anticipation adds to the excitement of getting head. Then you can try starting at the outer and inner lips.

- There are a couple ways to get the clit where you want it. The first is to press your nose into the area just above the clitoris at the apex of the labia majora (you will have to breathe through your mouth for this to work). This will cause the sweetest spot of the clit to pop out into your mouth. If she has a bit of a belly, place one hand there and push it upward toward her head. This will further position her clit right in your mouth. For the second technique, instead of pressing your nose above the clit, you can press your lips all the way around her clit, which stabilizes and helps stay on target, or use your thumb to press into the apex of the labia majora.

- Because all of the excess skin is out of the way, revealing the most sensitive part of the clit, it is not necessary to use long motions of the tongue but rather micro-movements in circles or up and down. Instead of using the tip of your tongue, use the flat, broad part for maximum contact (though sometimes the tip feels good too). Using this motion also causes less fatigue so you can last all the way through to orgasm. Start gentle and pay attention to what pressure brings her the most pleasure.

- Pussy eating is a job for the whole face. When done properly, your face, nose and chin will be wet. Use your whole face to melt into her vulva. If only your tongue is making contact with her vulva, you're not quite there yet.

- At this point she should be feeling immense pleasure. If she's not, adjust to her preference. Pay attention to your pressure because the most sensitive part of the clit will be exposed. Pressure is a tricky business. Too little will bring no pleasure. Too much will send her legs twitching and may not be pleasant (though she might not mind that). Check in with your partner to see how she is feeling.

- Women will often shift their hips to move you to the right spot. Pay attention. Let her.
- Incorporate the stimulation of other parts of the body, such as the vagina, anus or nipples.
- To be a great pussy-eater, you should definitely be incorporating the G-spot (forget about the debates around its existence). Have you ever said "Come here" with your fingers? If you do that inside the vagina, you will find the G-spot. With your partner on her back, insert your index and middle fingers knuckle-deep into the vagina, finger pads facing up. Curl your fingers up like you're saying "come here." She should like that. When you hit the G-spot, you are actually accessing the internal root of the clitoris and accompanying nerves. The external clit is just the tip of the iceberg, so to speak, and extends deeper within. You can also try inserting your fingers deeper within, using the same motion.
- Most women like it when you touch their nipples. Since they are very sensitive, this should be done with caution. However, if done too gently, it will not be very pleasurable. You can roll them between your fingers, gently pull them or suck them.

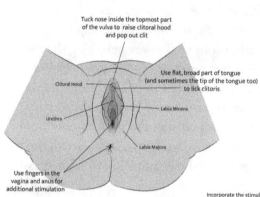

Tuck nose inside the topmost part of the vulva to raise clitoral hood and pop out clit

Use flat, broad part of tongue (and sometimes the tip of the tongue too) to lick clitoris

Clitoral Hood

Labia Minora

Urethra

Labia Majora

Use fingers in the vagina and anus for additional stimulation

Anatomy of the Vulva

Incorporate the stimulation of other parts of the body, such as the vagina, anus or nipples

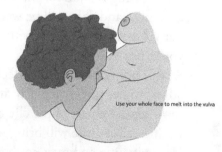

Use your whole face to melt into the vulva

Pussy-Eating Should Be an Experience for the Whole Face

- It can be very pleasurable for her while receiving head if you insert a finger into the anus, but ask first, because some people don't like this. You can use a moistened pinkie to start.

Hot Tips

- Remember that the female genitals, especially the clitoris, are very sensitive. Start gently, perhaps more gently than you think. Lots of women want to be licked harder though. If her clit gets stimulation overload, take a break or switch to licking the edges of the clit instead of the center. Others want you to stay right on the center of the clit the whole time. Just ask her what she's feeling.

- Let your partner know how much eating her out turns you on. This will be a big turn-on for her too.

- Repetition can be good. It can be really frustrating when a partner finally gets the right spot and then after thirty seconds they switch to something else. If she likes it, think about staying there.

- Different women respond to different things. The same woman may respond to different things on different days. Explore and have fun. Give yourself permission to grow. You might be bad at it at first, but practice makes perfect.

- You can use your lips to massage her clit in an up and down motion, similar to sucking a penis for variety. Some like it. Some don't. You can also suck on the inner lips and clit together.

- The tongue: It's common to use long lapping motions to lick the clitoris. This can be fatiguing and also difficult to stay on point, meaning the place which is most pleasurable. Using the tip of the tongue feels quite different than the flat part of it. You can incorporate both, according to your partner's preference. If you use the technique above to make the clit protrude into your mouth, you can use the flat center of your tongue to stay within a very small radius, honing in on the sweet spot of the clit for optimal pleasure.

- Tongue flick: rapid flicking of the clit with the tip of your tongue is highly pleasurable. Try different speeds and pressures. This is the most fatiguing though, so mix in other things. Switch from tip of tongue to the flat part, for example.

- Using these techniques should help keep your mouth and jaw from getting overly tired. But if they do, you can switch to using your fingers to stimulate the clitoris. Lots of women are happy to get off with just your hands. If you practice enough, you will be able to get just the right spot to bring her great pleasure while resting your neck and mouth. You can use circular or up-and-down motions with your fingers. Or you can insert your fingers into the vagina to access the G-spot while incorporating the thumb for clitoral stimulation. Try different speeds and pressures while communicating with her to see what she likes. Lube can often be helpful.

Oral sex can deepen intimacy in a partnership. With a little effort it can be intensely pleasurable for both the performer and the receiver. By humbling ourselves to learn what we don't know, we cultivate the beautiful art of giving. Best of all, it makes your partner feel adored by a very important person: you.

ACKNOWLEDGEMENTS

I would like to thank my family for their loving support, without which I could not have written this. In return, I continually gave them my vacant stare, as I was off in la la book land. Sorry about that.

Emily, you are a die-hard dreamer, a genius in the kitchen, and I can always count on your support. Thanks for dreaming with me. Thanks for your love Ellie, Harry, Jack, John, Sandy, Mom, Diane and Gary.

To my sister, Cori Hewett, thank you for being such a beautiful, kind person and for your appalling, inappropriate, filthy humor. Thanks for always making me feel normal.

Thank you so much to my exceptionally intelligent, clever, and funny editor, Tracy Moore. I am so glad that I persisted in my stalking efforts, tracking you down with very little information and getting you to take on this project. (Two former poor kids rocking the art of great sex!) You truly helped to breathe life into this book.

Thank you to Jeff "Mr. Pussy" Minerd for your hands-on approach to learning. And thank you to Chris Smith for the P.E. tutorial and all of your great tips. Thanks Daniel Maeso for the sex menu test kitchen.

Thank you Morgan Wittmer, the talented graphic artist who designed the cover, illustrations, and patiently indulged my constant indecision. Amie McCrackin, thanks for going above and beyond. Thanks John Paine for your editorial support. Thanks Bruno Álvarez for your exceptional Spanish translation of this book.

And last, but not least, thank you so much Bryan Isacks. You kindly (and freely) shared your TCM wisdom with me, even though you always first respond to my texts with "Who is this?"

About the Author

As an acupuncturist and herbalist in private practice, Christine DeLozier, L.Ac., specializes in sexual health, treating males, females, and all orientations and identities.

Acupuncture is great for sexual function, but to address the underlying mechanics of consistently great sex, diet is the key. For this reason, she works with patients to develop dietary habits that support their sexual goals.

Christine attended the University of Rochester, studying Biology and Psychology. As a young single mom, she worked as a waitress and studied full-time. She started in a program which trains students to be research scientists, but ultimately decided against a career in research. The experience, though, gave her an appreciation for the scientific method, which is employed throughout this book. She has exhaustively reviewed epidemiological and clinical research on nutrition and sexual function to shape the advice presented here.

Christine holds Master's degrees in Acupuncture, Traditional Chinese Medicine, and Counseling. During her education, she studied Chinese dietary therapy, and earned a certification as a Holistic Nutritional Counselor.

Early in her practice, she treated numerous men for erectile issues with acupuncture, who had significant improvements in sexual satisfaction. After seeing how meaningful this improvement was to their lives, she decided to specialize in sexual health, expanding her practice to all who seek it. She wanted to do more to help them connect with their partners and bring joy to their relationships. Since then she has treated adults looking to have great sex of all orientations.

Always rather obsessed with diet, nutrition, and natural health, Christine's philosophy is rooted in an evidence-based understanding of the physiological effect of food on the body, while honoring the wisdom of traditional Chinese medicine. She treats every patient holistically, as an individual and wishes to use her unique skill set to help others in a kind, loving way.

REFERENCES BY CHAPTER

Hormonal Balance and Great Sex

1   Ren Y, Yang X, Zhang Y, Wang Y, Li X. (2016). Effects and mechanisms of acupuncture and moxibustion on reproductive endocrine function in male rats with partial androgen deficiency. *Acupunct Med.* 2016;34(2):136-143.

2   Fu H, Sun J, Tan Y, et al. (2018). Effects of acupuncture on the levels of serum estradiol and pituitary estrogen receptor beta in a rat model of induced super ovulation. *Life Sci.* 2018;197:109-113.

3   Krysiak, R., Drosdzol-Cop, A., Skrzypulec-Plinta, V., & Okopien, B. (2016). Sexual function and depressive symptoms in young women with elevated macroprolactin content: a pilot study. *Endocrine,* 53(1), 291–298.

4   Araujo, A. B., & Wittert, G. A. (2011). Endocrinology of the aging male. Best practice & research. *Clinical endocrinology & metabolism,* 25(2), 303–319.

5   Anwar, Z., Sinha, V., Mitra, S., Mishra, A. K., Ansari, M. H., Bharti, A., Kumar, V., & Nigam, A. K. (2017). Erectile Dysfunction: An Underestimated Presentation in Patients with Diabetes Mellitus. *Indian journal of psychological medicine,* 39(5), 600–604.

6   Knoblovits, P. , Costanzo, P. R., Valzacchi, G. J., Gueglio, G. , Layus, A. O., Kozak, A. E., Balzaretti, M. I. and Litwak, L. E. (2010), Erectile Dysfunction, Obesity, Insulin Resistance, and Their Relationship With Testosterone Levels in Eugonadal Patients in an Andrology Clinic Setting. *Journal of Andrology,* 31: 263-270.

Eating to Balance Hormones

7   Franco-Pérez, J., Manjarrez-Marmolejo, J., Ballesteros-Zebadúa, P., Neri-Santos, A., Montes, S., Suarez-Rivera, N., Hernández-Cerón, M., & Pérez-Koldenkova, V. (2018). Chronic Consumption of Fructose Induces Behavioral Alterations by Increasing Orexin and Dopamine Levels in the Rat Brain. *Nutrients,* 10(11), 1722.

8   Vasconcelos, A. R., Cabral-Costa, J. V., Mazucanti, C. H., Scavone, C., & Kawamoto, E. M. (2016). The Role of Steroid Hormones in the Modulation of Neuroinflammation by Dietary Interventions. *Frontiers in endocrinology,* 7, 9.

9   Faulkner, L. D., Dowling, A. R., Stuart, R. C., Nillni, E. A., & Hill, J. W. (2015). Reduced melanocortin production causes sexual dysfunction in male mice with POMC neuronal insulin and leptin insensitivity. *Endocrinology,* 156(4), 1372–1385.

10 Franco-Pérez, J., Manjarrez-Marmolejo, J., Ballesteros-Zebadúa, P., Neri-Santos, A., Montes, S., Suarez-Rivera, N., Hernández-Cerón, M., & Pérez-Koldenkova, V. (2018). Chronic Consumption of Fructose Induces Behavioral Alterations by Increasing Orexin and Dopamine Levels in the Rat Brain. *Nutrients*, 10(11), 1722.

11 Schliep, K. C., Schisterman, E. F., Mumford, S. L., Pollack, A. Z., Perkins, N. J., Ye, A., Zhang, C. J., Stanford, J. B., Porucznik, C. A., Hammoud, A. O., & Wactawski-Wende, J. (2013). Energy-containing beverages: reproductive hormones and ovarian function in the BioCycle Study. *The American journal of clinical nutrition*, 97(3), 621–630.

12 Hatch, E. E., Wesselink, A. K., Hahn, K. A., Michiel, J. J., Mikkelsen, E. M., Sorensen, H. T., Rothman, K. J., & Wise, L. A. (2018). Intake of Sugar-sweetened Beverages and Fecundability in a North American Preconception Cohort. *Epidemiology* (Cambridge, Mass.), 29(3), 369–378.

13 Chen, L., Xie, Y. M., Pei, J. H., Kuang, J., Chen, H. M., Chen, Z., Li, Z. W., Fu, X. Y., Wang, L., Lai, S. Q., Zhang, S. T., Chen, Z. J., & Lin, J. X. (2018). Sugar-sweetened beverage intake and serum testosterone levels in adult males 20-39 years old in the United States. *Reproductive biology and endocrinology : RB&E*, 16(1), 61. https://doi.org/10.1186/s12958-018-0378-2

14 Aslankoc R, Ozmen O. (2019). The effects of high-fructose corn syrup consumption on testis physiopathology-The ameliorative role of melatonin. *Andrologia*. 2019;51(8):e13327.

15 Erlanson-Albertsson, C., & Albertsson, P. Å. (2015). The Use of Green Leaf Membranes to Promote Appetite Control, Suppress Hedonic Hunger and Loose Body Weight. *Plant foods for human nutrition* (Dordrecht, Netherlands), 70(3), 281–290.

16 Williams E.,Cabana F., Nekaris KAI. (2015). Improving Diet and Activity of Insectivorous Primates in Captivity: Naturalizing the Diet of Northern Ceylon Gray Slender Loris, Loris lydekkerianus nordicus. *Zoo Biology* 9999 : 1–10.

17 Milton, Katharine. (2006). Diet and Primate Evolution. *Scientific America, (June, 2006, 16, 3s) 22-29.*

18 Hamilton, W., & Busse, C. (1978). Primate Carnivory and Its Significance to Human Diets. *BioScience*, 28(12), 761-766.

19 Wayne SJ1, Neuhouser ML, Ulrich CM, Koprowski C, Baumgartner KB, Baumgartner RN, McTiernan A, Bernstein L, Ballard-Barbash R. (2008). Dietary fiber is associated with serum sex hormones and insulin-related peptides in postmenopausal breast cancer survivors.*Breast Cancer Res Treat.* Nov;112(1):149-58. Epub 2007 Dec 5.

20 Ghatei MA1, Ratcliffe B, Bloom SR, Goodlad RA.Fermentable dietary fibre, intestinal microflora and plasma hormones in the rat. *Clin Sci* (Lond). 1997 Aug;93(2):109-12.

21 Goldin BR., Adlercreutz H., Gorbach SL. (1982). Estrogen Excretion Patterns and Plasma Levels in Vegetarian and Omnivorous Women. *N Engl J Med* 1982; 307:1542-1547.

22 Cutler, D. A., Pride, S. M., & Cheung, A. P. (2019). Low intakes of dietary fiber and magnesium are associated with insulin resistance and hyperandrogenism in polycystic ovary syndrome: A cohort study. *Food science & nutrition*, 7(4), 1426–1437. doi:10.1002/fsn3.977

23 Zhong Y., Arumugam V., et al. (2015). Soluble dietary fiber (Fibersol-2) decreased hunger and increased satiety hormones in humans when ingested with a meal. *Nutrition Research*. Vol. 35, Issue 5. May 2015. P. 393-400.

24 Palacios, C., & Gonzalez, L. (2014). Is vitamin D deficiency a major global public health problem? *The Journal of steroid biochemistry and molecular biology*, 144 Pt A, 138–145.

25 Mann, M. C., Hollenberg, M. D., Hanley, D. A., & Ahmed, S. B. (2015). Vitamin D, the autonomic nervous system, and cardiovascular risk. Physiological reports, 3(4), e12349.

26 Sorenson, M., & Grant, W. B. (2012). Does vitamin D deficiency contribute to erectile dysfunction?. *Dermato-endocrinology*, 4(2), 128–136.

27 Zittermann A. (2013). Magnesium deficit overlooked cause of low vitamin D status? *BMC Med.* 2013;11229.

28   Cardwell, G., Bornman, J. F., James, A. P., & Black, L. J. (2018). A Review of Mushrooms as a Potential Source of Dietary Vitamin D. *Nutrients,* 10(10), 1498.

29   Navarro, S. L., Schwarz, Y., Song, X., Wang, C. Y., Chen, C., Trudo, S. P., Kristal, A. R., Kratz, M., Eaton, D. L., & Lampe, J. W. (2014). Cruciferous vegetables have variable effects on biomarkers of systemic inflammation in a randomized controlled trial in healthy young adults. *The Journal of nutrition,* 144(11), 1850–1857.

30   Hwang, C., Sethi, S., Heilbrun, L. K., Gupta, N. S., Chitale, D. A., Sakr, W. A., Menon, M., Peabody, J. O., Smith, D. W., Sarkar, F. H., & Heath, E. I. (2016). Anti-androgenic activity of absorption-enhanced 3, 3'-diindolylmethane in prostatectomy patients. *American journal of translational research,* 8(1), 166–176.

31   Lee, C. H., Jeong, S. J., Yun, S. M., Kim, J. H., Lee, H. J., Ahn, K. S., Won, S. H., Kim, H. S., Lee, H. J., Ahn, K. S., Zhu, S., Chen, C. Y., & Kim, S. H. (2010). Down-regulation of phosphoglucomutase 3 mediates sulforaphane-induced cell death in LNCaP prostate cancer cells. *Proteome science,* 8, 67.

32   Bernard G. Cipolla, Eric Mandron, Jean Marc Lefort, Yves Coadou, Emmanuel Della Negra, Luc Corbel, Ronan Le Scodan, Abdel Rahmene Azzouzi and Nicolas Mottet. (2015). Effect of Sulforaphane in Men with Biochemical Recurrence after Radical Prostatectomy. *Cancer Prev Res* August 1 2015 (8) (8) 712-719

33   Ma, T., Zhu, D., Chen, D., Zhang, Q., Dong, H., Wu, W., Lu, H., & Wu, G. (2018). Sulforaphane, a Natural Isothiocyanate Compound, Improves Cardiac Function and Remodeling by Inhibiting Oxidative Stress and Inflammation in a Rabbit Model of Chronic Heart Failure. *Medical science monitor : international medical journal of experimental and clinical research,* 24, 1473–1483.

34   Beklemisheva AA1, Feng J, Yeh YA, Wang LG, Chiao JW. (2007). Modulating testosterone stimulated prostate growth by phenethyl isothiocyanate via Sp1 and androgen receptor down-regulation. *Prostate.* 2007 Jun 1;67(8):863-70.

35   Huo, L., Su, Y., Xu, G., Zhai, L., & Zhao, J. (2019). Sulforaphane Protects the Male Reproductive System of Mice from Obesity-Induced Damage: Involvement of Oxidative Stress and Autophagy. *International journal of environmental research and public health,* 16(19), 3759.

36   Quirante-Moya S., García-Ibañez P., Quirante-Moya F., Villaño D., Moreno DA.(2020). Review: The Role of Brassica Bioactives on Human Health: Are We Studying It the Right Way? *Molecules.* March 2020.

37   Calderón-Ospina, C. A., & Nava-Mesa, M. O. (2020). B Vitamins in the nervous system: Current knowledge of the biochemical modes of action and synergies of thiamine, pyridoxine, and cobalamin. *CNS neuroscience & therapeutics,* 26(1), 5–13.

38   Ishibashi S, Yokota T, Shiojiri T, Matunaga T, Tanaka H, Nishina K, Hirota H, Inaba A, Yamada M, Kanda T, Mizusawa H. (2003). Reversible acute axonal polyneuropathy associated with Wernicke-Korsakoff syndrome: impaired physiological nerve conduction due to thiamine deficiency? *J Neurol Neurosurg Psychiatry.* 74:674–676

39   H.L. Hernández-Montiel, C.M. Vásquez López, J.G. González-Loyola. (2014). Chronic administration of thiamine pyrophosphate decreases age-related histological atrophic testicular changes and improves sexual behavior in male Wistar rats. *Histol Histopathol.* 2014 Jun;29(6):785-95. doi: 10.14670/HH-29.785. Epub 2013 Dec 20

40   Suwannasom, N., Kao, I., Pruß, A., Georgieva, R., & Bäumler, H. (2020). Riboflavin: The Health Benefits of a Forgotten Natural Vitamin. *International journal of molecular sciences,* 21(3), 950.

41   M. W. Esch, R. A. Easter, J. M. Bahr. (1981). Effect of Riboflavin Deficiency on Estrous Cyclicity in Pigs. *Biology of Reproduction,* Volume 25, Issue 3, 1 October 1981, Pages 659–665

42 Shomali T, Taherianfard M, Dalvand M, Namazi F. (2018). Effect of pharmacological doses of niacin on testicular structure and function in normal and diabetic rats. *Andrologia*. 2018 Dec;50(10):e13142. doi: 10.1111/and.13142. Epub 2018 Sep 6.

43 Ng CF, Lee CP, Ho AL, Lee VW. (2011). Effect of niacin on erectile function in men suffering erectile dysfunction and dyslipidemia. J *Sex Med*. 2011 Oct;8(10):2883-93.

44 Yamamoto T., Jaroenporn S., Pan L., et al. (2009). Effects of pantothenic acid on testicular function in male rats. *J Vet Med Sci*. 2009 Nov;71(11):1427-32.

45 Jolivalt CG, Mizisin LM, Nelson A, Cunha JM, Ramos KM, Bonke D, Calcutt NA.(2009). B vitamins alleviate indices of neuropathic pain in diabetic rats. *Eur J Pharmacol*. 2009 Jun 10;612(1-3):41-7.

46 Symes EK, Bender DA, Bowden JF, Coulson WF. (1984). Increased target tissue uptake of, and sensitivity to, testosterone in the vitamin B6 deficient rat. *J Steroid Biochem*. 1984 May;20(5):1089-93.

47 Sansone M, Sansone A, Romano M, Seraceno S, Di Luigi L, Romanelli F. (2018). Folate: a possible role in erectile dysfunction? *Aging Male*. 2018 Jun;21(2):116-120.

48 Yan, W. J., Yu, N., Yin, T. L., Zou, Y. J., & Yang, J. (2014). A new potential risk factor in patients with erectile dysfunction and premature ejaculation: folate deficiency. *Asian journal of andrology*, 16(6), 902–906.

49 Mottaghi T, Khorvash F, Maracy M, Bellissimo N & Askari G. (2019). Effect of folic acid supplementation on nerve conduction velocity in diabetic polyneuropathy patients. *Neurological Research*, 41:4, 364-368, DOI: 10.1080/01616412.2019.1565180

50 Leishear, K., Boudreau, R. M., Studenski, S. A., Ferrucci, L., Rosano, C., de Rekeneire, N., Houston, D. K., Kritchevsky, S. B., Schwartz, A. V., Vinik, A. I., Hogervorst, E., Yaffe, K., Harris, T. B., Newman, A. B., Strotmeyer, E. S., & Health, Aging and Body Composition Study (2012). Relationship between vitamin B12 and sensory and motor peripheral nerve function in older adults. *Journal of the American Geriatrics Society*, 60(6), 1057–1063.

51 Kim K, Mills JL, Michels KA, et al. (2020). Dietary Intakes of Vitamin B-2 (Riboflavin), Vitamin B-6, and Vitamin B-12 and Ovarian Cycle Function among Premenopausal Women. *J Acad Nutr Diet*. 2020 May;120(5):885-892.

52 Obersby D, Chappell DC, Dunnett A, Tsiami AA. (2013). Plasma total homocysteine status of vegetarians compared with omnivores: a systematic review and meta-analysis. *Br J Nutr*. 2013 Mar 14;109(5):785-94.

53 Leishear, K., Boudreau, R. M., Studenski, S. A., Ferrucci, L., Rosano, C., de Rekeneire, N., Houston, D. K., Kritchevsky, S. B., Schwartz, A. V., Vinik, A. I., Hogervorst, E., Yaffe, K., Harris, T. B., Newman, A. B., Strotmeyer, E. S., & Health, Aging and Body Composition Study (2012). Relationship between vitamin B12 and sensory and motor peripheral nerve function in older adults. *Journal of the American Geriatrics Society*, 60(6), 1057–1063.

54 Fujii A1, Matsumoto H, Yamamoto H.(1996). Effect of vitamin B complex on neurotransmission and neurite outgrowth. *Gen Pharmacol*. 1996 Sep;27(6):995-1000.

55 Banihani S. A. (2017). Vitamin B12 and Semen Quality. *Biomolecules*, 7(2), 42.

56 Green, R., Allen, L., Bjørke-Monsen, A. et al. (2017). Vitamin B12 deficiency. *Nat Rev Dis Primers* 3, 17040

57 Mattson, M. P., Longo, V. D., & Harvie, M. (2017). Impact of intermittent fasting on health and disease processes. *Ageing research reviews*, 39, 46–58.

58 Anton, S. D., Moehl, K., Donahoo, W. T., Marosi, K., Lee, S. A., Mainous, A. G., 3rd, Leeuwenburgh, C., & Mattson, M. P. (2018). Flipping the Metabolic Switch: Understanding and Applying the Health Benefits of Fasting. *Obesity* (Silver Spring, Md.), 26(2), 254–268.

59 Golbidi, Saeid & Daiber, Andreas & Korac, Bato & Li, Huige & Essop, M Faadiel & Laher, Ismail. (2017). Health Benefits of Fasting and Caloric Restriction. *Current Diabetes Reports*. 17. 10.1007/s11892-017-0951-7.

60   Nair, P. M., & Khawale, P. G. (2016). Role of therapeutic fasting in women's health: An overview. *Journal of mid-life health*, 7(2), 61–64

61   Longo, V. D., & Mattson, M. P. (2014). Fasting: molecular mechanisms and clinical applications. *Cell metabolism*, 19(2), 181–192.

62   Nair, P. M., & Khawale, P. G. (2016). Role of therapeutic fasting in women's health: An overview. *Journal of mid-life health*, 7(2), 61–64.

63   Mattison JA1, Lane MA, Roth GS, Ingram DK.Calorie restriction in rhesus monkeys. *Exp Gerontol*. 2003 Jan-Feb;38(1-2):35-46.

64   Martin, B., Pearson, M., Kebejian, L., Golden, E., Keselman, A., Bender, M., Carlson, O., Egan, J., Ladenheim, B., Cadet, J. L., Becker, K. G., Wood, W., Duffy, K., Vinayakumar, P., Maudsley, S., & Mattson, M. P. (2007). Sex-dependent metabolic, neuroendocrine, and cognitive responses to dietary energy restriction and excess. *Endocrinology*, 148(9), 4318–4333.

65   Martin, C. K., Bhapkar, M., Pittas, A. G., Pieper, C. F., Das, S. K., Williamson, D. A., Scott, T., Redman, L. M., Stein, R., Gilhooly, C. H., Stewart, T., Robinson, L., Roberts, S. B., & Comprehensive Assessment of Long-term Effects of Reducing Intake of Energy (CALERIE) Phase 2 Study Group (2016). Effect of Calorie Restriction on Mood, Quality of Life, Sleep, and Sexual Function in Healthy Nonobese Adults: The CALERIE 2 Randomized Clinical Trial. *JAMA internal medicine*, 176(6), 743–752.

66   Martin, B., Pearson, M., Brenneman, R., Golden, E., Wood, W., Prabhu, V., Becker, K. G., Mattson, M. P., & Maudsley, S. (2009). Gonadal transcriptome alterations in response to dietary energy intake: sensing the reproductive environment. *PloS one*, 4(1), e4146.

67   Ho, K. Y., Veldhuis, J. D., Johnson, M. L., Furlanetto, R., Evans, W. S., Alberti, K. G., & Thorner, M. O. (1988). Fasting enhances growth hormone secretion and amplifies the complex rhythms of growth hormone secretion in man. *The Journal of clinical investigation*, 81(4), 968–975.

68   Patterson, R. E., Laughlin, G. A., LaCroix, A. Z., Hartman, S. J., Natarajan, L., Senger, C. M., Martínez, M. E., Villaseñor, A., Sears, D. D., Marinac, C. R., & Gallo, L. C. (2015). Intermittent Fasting and Human Metabolic Health. *Journal of the Academy of Nutrition and Dietetics*, 115(8), 1203–1212.

69   Roth GS1, Handy AM, Mattison JA, Tilmont EM, Ingram DK, Lane MA.(2002). Effects of dietary caloric restriction and aging on thyroid hormones of rhesus monkeys. *Horm Metab Res*. 2002 Jul;34(7):378-82.

70   Cangemi, R., Friedmann, A. J., Holloszy, J. O., & Fontana, L. (2010). Long-term effects of calorie restriction on serum sex-hormone concentrations in men. *Aging cell*, 9(2), 236–242.

The Nervous System and Great Sex

71   Sipski, M.L. (2002). Central Nervous System Based Neurogenic Female Sexual Dysfunction: Current Status and Future Trends. *Arch Sex Behav* 31: 421.

72   Azadzoi, KM, Siroky, MB. (2010). Neurologic Factors in Female Sexual Function and Dysfunction. *Korean J Urol*. Jul; 51(7): 443–449

73   Valles-Antuña, C., Fernandez-Gomez, J. and Fernandez-Gonzalez, F. (2011), Peripheral neuropathy: an underdiagnosed cause of erectile dysfunction. *BJU International*. 108: 1855-1859

74   Garcia de Gurtubay Galligo I, Morales Blanquez G, Navajas Carasa D et al. (1999). Neurophysiologic Techniques in the Diagnosis of Erectile Dysfunction: Study of 105 Cases. *Arch Esplanade's Urol*. Apr;52(3):262-8

75 Cortelazzi D1, Marconi A, Guazzi M, et al (2013). Sexual dysfunction in pre-menopausal diabetic women: clinical, metabolic, psychological, cardiovascular, and neurophysiologic correlates. *Acta Diabetol.* Dec;50(6):911-7

76 Li, H., Jiang, H., & Liu, J. (2017). Traditional Chinese medical therapy for erectile dysfunction. *Translational andrology and urology.* 6(2), 192–198.

77 Palve, S. S., & Palve, S. B. (2018). Impact of Aging on Nerve Conduction Velocities and Late Responses in Healthy Individuals. *Journal of neurosciences in rural practice.* 9(1), 112–116.

78 Lauretani, F., Bandinelli, S., Bartali, B., et al (2007). Omega-6 and omega-3 fatty acids predict accelerated decline of peripheral nerve function in older persons. *European journal of neurology.* 14(7), 801–808.

79 Mrakic-Sposta, S., Vezzoli, A., Maderna, L., et al. (2018). R(+)-Thioctic Acid Effects on Oxidative Stress and Peripheral Neuropathy in Type II Diabetic Patients: Preliminary Results by Electron Paramagnetic Resonance and Electroneurography. *Oxidative medicine and cellular longevity.* 1767265.

80 Jabeen A., Khan UA., Ayub M., Hameed MA.(2011). Effects of simvastatin and alpha-tocopherol on disturbed nerve conduction in obese Sprague Dawley rats. *J Ayub Med Coll Abbottabad.* Jul-Sep;23(3):18-22.

81 Asadi, N., Bahmani, M., Kheradmand, A., & Rafieian-Kopaei, M. (2017). The Impact of Oxidative Stress on Testicular Function and the Role of Antioxidants in Improving it: A Review. Journal of clinical and diagnostic research : JCDR, 11(5), IE01–IE05.

82 Erdman J, Balentine D, Arab L, Beecher G, Dwyer J, Folts J, Harnly J, Hollman P, Keen C, Mazza et al. (2005). Flavonoids and Heart Health: Proceedings of the ILSI North America Flavonoids Workshop, May 31–June 1, 2005, Washington, DC. *Journal of Nutrition.* Volume 137, Issue 3. March 2007. Bondonna C, Yang X, Croft KD, Considine MJ, Ward NC, Rich L, Puddy IB, Swinny E, Mubarak A, Hodgson JM. (2012). Flavonoid-rich apples and nitrate-rich spinach augment nitric oxide status and improve endothelial function in healthy men and women: a randomized controlled trial. *Free Radical Biology and Medicine.* Volume 52, Issue 1, 1 January, Pages 95-102 Lewicka M, Henrykowska G, Zawadzka M, Rutkowski M, Pacholski K, Buczyński A. (2017).
Impact of electromagnetic radiation emitted by monitors on changes in the cellular membrane   structure and protective antioxidant effect of vitamin A - In vitro study. *Int J Occup Med Environ   Health.* 2017 Jul 14;30(5):695-703 Pérez-Cano FJ, Castell M. (2016). Flavonoids, Inflammation and Immune System. *Nutrients.* 8(10):659 · October 2016

83 Islam MW., Tariq M., Ageel AM., al-Said MS., al-Yhya AM. (1991). Effect of Salvia haematodes on sexual behaviour of male rats. J *Ethnopharmacol.* May-Jun;33(1-2):67-72.

84 Chen, CY., Li, H., Yuan, YN., et al.(2013). Antioxidant activity and components of a traditional Chinese medicine formula consisting of Crataegus pinnatifida and Salvia miltiorrhiza. *BMC complementary and alternative medicine.*13, 99.

85 Bondonna C, Yang X, Croft KD, Considine MJ, Ward NC, Rich L, Puddy IB, Swinny E, Mubarak A, Hodgson JM. (2012). Flavonoid-rich apples and nitrate-rich spinach augment nitric oxide status and improve endothelial function in healthy men and women: a randomized controlled trial. Free Radical Biology and Medicine. Volume 52, Issue 1, 1 January, Pages 95-102

Mushrooms, Nerves and Great Sex

86 Lindequist, U., Niedermeyer, T. H., & Jülich, W. D. (2005). The pharmacological potential of mushrooms. *Evidence-based complementary and alternative medicine: eCAM,* 2(3), 285–299.

87   de Groot, P. F., Frissen, M. N., de Clercq, N. C., & Nieuwdorp, M. (2017). Fecal microbiota transplantation in metabolic syndrome: History, present and future. *Gut microbes,* 8(3), 253–267.

88   Dominguez-Bello, M. G., De Jesus-Laboy, K. M., Shen, N.et al (2016). Partial restoration of the microbiota of cesarean-born infants via vaginal microbial transfer. *Nature medicine.* 22(3), 250–253.

89   Neu, J., Rushing, J. (2011). Cesarean versus vaginal delivery: long-term infant outcomes and the hygiene hypothesis. *Clinics in perinatology.* 38(2), 321–331.

90   Murphy EF, Cotter PD, Healy S, Marques TM, O'Sullivan O, Fouhy F, Clarke SF, O'Toole PW, Quigley EM, Stanton C, Ross PR, O'Doherty RM, Shanahan F. (2010). Composition and energy harvesting capacity of the gut microbiota: relationship to diet, obesity and time in mouse models. *Gut.* 2010, 59 (12): 1635-1642.

91   Nelson AM, Walk ST, Taube S, Taniuchi M, Houpt ER, Wobus CE, Young VB. (2012). Disruption of the human gut microbiota following Norovirus infection. *PLoS One.* 2012, 7 (10): e48224-

92   Perez-Cobas AE, Gosalbes MJ, Friedrichs A, Knecht H, Artacho A, Eismann K, Otto W, Rojo D, Bargiela R, Von Bergen M, von Bergen M, Neulinger SC, Daumer C, Heinsen FA, Latorre A, Barbas C, Seifert J, Dos Santos VM, Ott SJ, Ferrer M, Moya A. (2012). Gut microbiota disturbance during antibiotic therapy: a multi-omic approach. Gut. 2012

93   Petriz, B.A., Castro, A.P., Almeida, J.A. et al. (2014). Exercise induction of gut microbiota modifications in obese, non-obese and hypertensive rats. *BMC Genomics* 15, 511

94   Santacruz A, Marcos A, Warnberg J, Marti A, Martin-Matillas M, Campoy C, Moreno LA, Veiga O, Redondo-Figuero C, Garagorri JM, Azcona C, Delgado M, Garcia-Fuentes M, Collado MC, Sanz Y. (2009). Interplay between weight loss and gut microbiota composition in overweight adolescents. *Obesity* (Silver Spring). 2009, 17 (10): 1906-1915.

95   Sharon G., Sampson T. R., Geschwind, D. H., & Mazmanian, S. K. (2016). The Central Nervous System and the Gut Microbiome. *Cell.* 167(4), 915–932.

96   Tirandaz H, Bagher M, Borhan M, Raoofi S, Ebrahim H. (2018). Microbiota Potential for the Treatment of Sexual Dysfunction. *Medical Hypotheses.* 115. 46-49.

97   Pallav K., Dowd S.E., Villafuerte J., et al. (2014). Effects of polysaccharopeptide from Trametes versicolor and amoxicillin on the gut microbiome of healthy volunteers. *Gut Microbes.* 5:458–467.

98   Jayachandran, M., Xiao, J., & Xu, B. (2017). A Critical Review on Health Promoting Benefits of Edible Mushrooms through Gut Microbiota. *International journal of molecular sciences.* 18(9), 1934.

99   Yu, S., Weaver, V., Martin, K., & Cantorna, M. T. (2009). The effects of whole mushrooms during inflammation. *BMC immunology.* 10, 12.

100   Varshney, J., Ooi, J. H., Jayarao, B. M., Albert, I., Fisher, J., Smith, R. L., Patterson, A. D., & Cantorna, M. T. (2013). White button mushrooms increase microbial diversity and accelerate the resolution of Citrobacter rodentium infection in mice. *The Journal of nutrition.* 143(4), 526–532.

101   Trovato Salinaro, A., Pennisi, M., Di Paola, R.et al. (2018). Neuroinflammation and neurohormesis in the pathogenesis of Alzheimer's disease and Alzheimer-linked pathologies: modulation by nutritional mushrooms. *Immunity & ageing : I & A,* 15, 8.

102   Samberkar S., Gandhi S., Sivasangkary N., et al. (2016). Lion's Mane, Hericium erinaceus and Tiger Milk, Lignosus rhinocerotis (Higher Basidiomycetes) Medicinal Mushrooms Stimulate Neurite Outgrowth in Dissociated Cells of Brain, Spinal Cord, and Retina: An In Vitro Study. *International Journal of Medicinal Mushrooms.* 17. 10.1615

103   Kah Hui, Wong & Ng, Chai-Chee & Kanagasabapathy, Gowri & Yow, Yoon-Yen & Sabaratnam, Vikineswary. (2017). An Overview of Culinary and Medicinal Mushrooms in Neurodegeneration and Neurotrauma Research. *International Journal of Medicinal Mushrooms.* 19. 191-202. 10.1615/

104   Okolo, K. O., Siminialayi, I. M., & Orisakwe, O. E. (2016). Protective Effects of Pleurotus tuber-regium on Carbon- Tetrachloride Induced Testicular Injury in Sprague Dawley Rats. *Frontiers in pharmacology.* 7, 480.

105   Valverde, M. E., Hernández-Pérez, T., & Paredes-López, O. (2015). Edible mushrooms: improving human health and promoting quality life. *International journal of microbiology.* 2015, 376387

106   Chang, C. J., Lin, C. S., Lu, C. C., et al (2015). Ganoderma lucidum reduces obesity in mice by modulating the composition of the gut microbiota. *Nature communications.* 6, 7489.

107   APA Chang, C. J., Lin, C. S., Lu, C. et al. (2015). Ganoderma lucidum reduces obesity in mice by modulating the composition of the gut microbiota. *Nature communications.* 6, 7489.

108   Chen, J., Jin, X., Zhang, L., & Yang, L. (2013). A study on the antioxidant effect of Coriolus versicolor polysaccharide in rat brain tissues. *African journal of traditional, complementary, and alternative medicines.*10(6), 481–484.

109   Ferreiro, E., Pita, I. R., Mota, S. I.,et al. (2018). Coriolus versicolor biomass increases dendritic arborization of newly-generated neurons in mouse hippocampal dentate gyrus. *Oncotarget.* 9(68), 32929–32942.

110   Ho, C. S., Tung, Y. T., Kung, et al. (2017). Effect of Coriolus versicolor Mycelia Extract on Exercise Performance and Physical Fatigue in Mice. *International journal of medical sciences.* 14(11), 1110–1117.

111   Palacios, S., Losa, F., Dexeus, D., & Cortés, J. (2017). Beneficial effects of a Coriolus versicolor-based vaginal gel on cervical epithelization, vaginal microbiota and vaginal health: a pilot study in asymptomatic women. *BMC women's health.* 17(1), 21.

112   Wong, K. H., Naidu, M., David, P., et al. (2011). Peripheral Nerve Regeneration Following Crush Injury to Rat Peroneal Nerve by Aqueous Extract of Medicinal Mushroom Hericium erinaceus (Bull.: Fr) Pers. (Aphyllophoromycetideae). *Evidence-based complementary and alternative medicine:* eCAM, 2011, 580752.

113   Nagai, K., Chiba, A., Nishino, T., Kubota, T., & Kawagishi, H. (2006). Dilinoleoyl-phosphatidylethanolamine from Hericium erinaceum protects against ER stress-dependent Neuro2a cell death via protein kinase C pathway. *Journal of Nutritional Biochemistry.*17(8), 525–530.

114   Sabaratnam, V., Kah-Hui, W., Naidu, M., & Rosie David, P. (2013). Neuronal health - can culinary and medicinal mushrooms help?. *Journal of traditional and complementary medicine,* 3(1), 62–68.

115   Jiraungkoorskul, K., & Jiraungkoorskul, W. (2016). Review of Naturopathy of Medical Mushroom, Ophiocordyceps Sinensis, in Sexual Dysfunction. *Pharmacognosy reviews,* 10(19), 1–5.

116   Dotan N1, Wasser SP, Mahajna J. (2011). The culinary-medicinal mushroom Coprinus comatus as a natural antiandrogenic modulator. *Integr Cancer Ther.* 2011 Jun;10(2):148-59.

117   Dotan N1, Wasser SP, Mahajna J. (2011). The culinary-medicinal mushroom Coprinus comatus as a natural antiandrogenic modulator. *Integr Cancer Ther.* 2011 Jun;10(2):148-59.

118   Rossi, P., Buonocore, D., Altobelli, E., et al. (2014). Improving Training Condition Assessment in Endurance Cyclists: Effects of Ganoderma lucidum and Ophiocordyceps sinensis Dietary Supplementation. *Evidence-based complementary and alternative medicine* : eCAM, 2014, 979613.

119   Yoo Kyoung Park Hyang Burm Lee Eun-Jae Jeon Hack Sung Jung Myung-Hee Kang (2008). Chaga mushroom extract inhibits oxidative DNA damage in human lymphocytes as assessed by comet assay. *Biofactors*.21(1-4):109-12.

The Vascular System and Great Sex

120   Liu AH, Bondonno CP, Croft KD, Puddey IB, Woodman RJ, Rich L, Ward NC, Vita JA, Hodgson JM. (2013). Effects of a nitrate-rich meal on arterial stiffness and blood pressure in healthy volunteers. *Nitric Oxide* Volume 35, 30 November 2013, Pages 123-130

121   Esselstyn C. B. (2017). A plant-based diet and coronary artery disease: a mandate for effective therapy. *Journal of geriatric cardiology*: JGC, 14(5), 317–320. doi:10.11909/j.issn.1671-5411.2017.05.004

122   Munarriz R1, Kim SW, Kim NN, Traish A, Goldstein I. (2003). A review of the physiology and pharmacology of peripheral (vaginal and clitoral) female genital arousal in the animal model. *J Urol.* 2003 Aug;170(2 Pt 2):S40-4; discussion S44-5.

123   Berman JR1, Berman LA, Toler SM, Gill J, Haughie S; Sildenafil Study Group. (2003). Safety and efficacy of sildenafil citrate for the treatment of female sexual arousal disorder: a double-blind, placebo controlled study. *J Urol.* 2003 Dec;170(6 Pt 1):2333-8.

124   Herlihy, L. K., Walsh, D. M., Burke, E., Crowley, V., & Mahmud, A. (2013). Postprandial effect of dietary fat quantity and quality on arterial stiffness and wave reflection: a randomised controlled trial. *Nutrition journal,* 12, 93

125   Lithander, F. E., Herlihy, L. K., Walsh, D. M., Burke, E., Crowley, V., & Mahmud, A. (2013). Postprandial effect of dietary fat quantity and quality on arterial stiffness and wave reflection: a randomised controlled trial. *Nutrition journal,* 12, 93 Nicholls SJ1, Lundman P, Harmer JA, Cutri B, Griffiths KA, Rye KA, Barter PJ, Celermajer DS.(2006). Consumption of saturated fat impairs the anti-inflammatory properties of high-density lipoproteins and endothelial function. *J Am Coll Cardiol.* Aug 15;48(4):715-20

126   Esposito K1, Ciotola M, Maiorino MI, Giugliano F, Autorino R, De Sio M, Cozzolino D, Saccomanno F, Giugliano D.(2009). Hyperlipidemia and sexual function in premenopausal women. *J Sex Med.* 2009 Jun;6(6):1696-1703.

127   Chakraborty, T. R., Donthireddy, L., Adhikary, D., & Chakraborty, S. (2016). Long-Term High Fat Diet Has a Profound Effect on Body Weight, Hormone Levels, and Estrous Cycle in Mice. *Medical science monitor : international medical journal of experimental and clinical research,* 22, 1601–1608.

128   Huang YC, Ho DR, Lin JH, Huang KT, Chen CS, Shi CS. Dietary Modification Is Associated with Normalization of Penile Hemodynamics in Rats Fed a High-Fat Diet. *J Sex Med.* 2019 Jun;16(6):791-802.

129   Randrup E, Baum N, Feibus A. (2015) Erectile dysfunction and cardiovascular disease, *Postgraduate Medicine,* 127:2, 166-172,

130   Hannan, J. L., Cheung, G. L., Blaser, M. C., Pang, J. J., Pang, S. C., Webb, R. C., & Adams, M. A. (2012). Characterization of the vasculature supplying the genital tissues in female rats. *The journal of sexual medicine,* 9(1), 136–147.

131   Diaconu CC, Manea M, Marcu DR, Socea B, Spinu AD, Bratu OG. The erectile dysfunction as a marker of cardiovascular disease: a review. *Acta Cardiol.* 2019 Apr 6:1-7.

132   Meldrum DR, Gambone JC, Morris MA, Meldrum DA, Esposito K, Ignarro LJ. The link between erectile and cardiovascular health: the canary in the coal mine. *Am J Cardiol.* 2011 Aug 15; 108(4):599-606. Epub 2011 May 31.

133   Inman, B. A., Sauver, J. L., Jacobson, D. J., McGree, M. E., Nehra, A., Lieber, M. M., ... Jacobsen, S. J. (2009). A population-based, longitudinal study of erectile dysfunction and future coronary artery disease. *Mayo Clinic proceedings,* 84(2), 108–113.

134   APA Vasconcelos, A. R., Cabral-Costa, J. V., Mazucanti, C. H., Scavone, C., & Kawamoto, E. M. (2016). The Role of Steroid Hormones in the Modulation of Neuroinflammation by Dietary Interventions. *Frontiers in endocrinology,* 7, 9.

135   Ornish D, Scherwitz LW, Billings JH, et al. Intensive Lifestyle Changes for Reversal of Coronary Heart Disease. *JAMA.* 1998;280(23):2001–2007

136   Esselstyn CB Jr1, Ellis SG, Medendorp SV, Crowe (1995). A strategy to arrest and reverse coronary artery disease: a 5-year longitudinal study of a single physician's practice. *TD.J Fam Pract.* Dec;41(6):560-8.

137   Dimina L, Mariotti F. (2019). Review: The Postprandial Appearance of Features of Cardiometabolic Risk: Acute Induction and Prevention by Nutrients and Other Dietary Substances. Nutrients. 11(9), 1963

138   Liu, A. G., Ford, N. A., Hu, F. B., Zelman, K. M., Mozaffarian, D., & Kris-Etherton, P. M. (2017). A healthy approach to dietary fats: understanding the science and taking action to reduce consumer confusion. *Nutrition journal,* 16(1), 53.

139   Mumford, S. L., Chavarro, J. E., Zhang, C., Perkins, N. J., Sjaarda, L. A., Pollack, A. Z., Schliep, K. C., Michels, K. A., Zarek, S. M., Plowden, T. C., Radin, R. G., Messer, L. C., Frankel, R. A., & Wactawski-Wende, J. (2016). Dietary fat intake and reproductive hormone concentrations and ovulation in regularly menstruating women. *The American journal of clinical nutrition,* 103(3), 868–877.

140   Young G1, Conquer J. (2005). Omega-3 fatty acids and neuropsychiatric disorders. *Reprod Nutr Dev.* Jan-Feb;45(1):1-28.

141   Graf, H., Malejko, K., Metzger, C. D., Walter, M., Grön, G., & Abler, B. (2019). Serotonergic, Dopaminergic, and Noradrenergic Modulation of Erotic Stimulus Processing in the Male Human Brain. *Journal of clinical medicine,* 8(3), 363.

142   Ross, B. M., Seguin, J., & Sieswerda, L. E. (2007). Omega-3 fatty acids as treatments for mental illness: which disorder and which fatty acid?. *Lipids in health and disease,* 6, 21.

143   McNamara, R. K., Able, J., Jandacek, R., Rider, T., & Tso, P. (2009). Gender differences in rat erythrocyte and brain docosahexaenoic acid composition: role of ovarian hormones and dietary omega-3 fatty acid composition. 34(4), 532–539. https://doi.org/10.1016/j.psyneuen.2008.10.013

144   Barros, M. P., Poppe, S. C., & Bondan, E. F. (2014). Neuroprotective properties of the marine carotenoid astaxanthin and omega-3 fatty acids, and perspectives for the natural combination of both in krill oil. *Nutrients,* 6(3), 1293–1317.

145   Delattre AM, Kiss A, Szawka RE, et al. (2010). Evaluation of chronic omega-3 fatty acids supplementation on behavioral and neurochemical alterations in 6-hydroxydopamine-lesion model of Parkinson's disease. *Neurosci Res.* Mar;66(3):256-64.

146   Ko GD., Nowacki NB., Arseneau L., Eitel M., Hum A. (2010). Omega-3 fatty acids for neuropathic pain: case series. *Clin J Pain.* Feb;26(2):168-72

147   Stockard J.E., Saste M.D., Benford V.J., et al. (2000). Effect of Docosahexaenoic Acid Content of Maternal Diet on Auditory Brainstem Conduction Times in Rat Pups. *Dev Neurosci.* 22:494–499

148   Lauretani, F., Bandinelli, S., Bartali, B., Cherubini, A., Iorio, A. D., Blè, A., ... Ferrucci, L. (2007). Omega-6 and omega-3 fatty acids predict accelerated decline of peripheral nerve function in older persons. *European journal of neurology,* 14(7), 801–808.

149 Patten GS, Abeywardena MY, McMurchie EJ, Jahangiri A. (2002). Dietary Fish Oil Increases Acetylcholine- and Eicosanoid-Induced Contractility of Isolated Rat Ileum, *The Journal of Nutrition.* Volume 132, Issue 9, 2506–2513

150 Nehra, D., Le, H. D., Fallon, E. M., Carlson, et al. (2012). Prolonging the female reproductive lifespan and improving egg quality with dietary omega-3 fatty acids. *Aging cell,* 11(6), 1046–1054.

151 Mumford, S. L., Chavarro, J. E., Zhang, C., Perkins, N. J., Sjaarda, L. A., Pollack, A. Z., Schliep, K. C., Michels, K. A., Zarek, S. M., Plowden, T. C., Radin, R. G., Messer, L. C., Frankel, R. A., & Wactawski-Wende, J. (2016). Dietary fat intake and reproductive hormone concentrations and ovulation in regularly menstruating women. *The American journal of clinical nutrition,* 103(3), 868–877.

152 Liao, C. H., Wu, Y. N., Chen, B. H., Lin, Y. H., Ho, H. O., & Chiang, H. S. (2016). Neuroprotective effect of docosahexaenoic acid nanoemulsion on erectile function in a rat model of bilateral cavernous nerve injury. *Scientific reports,* 6, 33040.

153 MInguez-Alarcón, L., Chavarro, J. E., Mendiola, J., Roca, M., Tanrikut, C., Vioque, J., Jørgensen, N., & Torres-Cantero, A. M. (2017). Fatty acid intake in relation to reproductive hormones and testicular volume among young healthy men. *Asian journal of andrology,* 19(2), 184–190.

Minerals

154 Murawski M, Bydłoń G, Sawicka-Kapusta K, Wierzchoś E, Zakrzewska M, Włodarczyk S, Molik E, Zieba D (2006).The effect of long term exposure to copper on physiological condition and reproduction of sheep.*Reprod Biol.* 2006; 6 Suppl 1():201-6.

155 Kim, K., Wactawski-Wende, J., Michels, K. A., Schliep, K. C., Plowden, T. C., Chaljub, E. N., & Mumford, S. L. (2018). Dietary minerals, reproductive hormone levels and sporadic anovulation: associations in healthy women with regular menstrual cycles. The *British journal of nutrition,* 120(1), 81–89.

156 Ruder EH, Hartman TJ, Goldman MB. (2009). Impact of oxidative stress on female fertility. *Curr Opin Obstet Gynecol.* 2009;21(3):219-222.

157 Cogswell ME1, Zhang Z, Carriquiry AL, Gunn JP, Kuklina EV, Saydah SH, Yang Q, Moshfegh AJ.(2012). Sodium and potassium intakes among US adults: NHANES 2003-2008. *Am J Clin Nutr.* 2012 Sep;96(3):647-57

158 Oberleithner, H., Riethmüller, C., Schillers, H., Macgregor, G.A., Wardener, H.E., & Hausberg, M. (2007). Plasma sodium stiffens vascular endothelium and reduces nitric oxide release. Proceedings of the National Academy of Sciences of the United States of America, 104 41, 16281-6 .

159 Frassetto, Lynda & Morris, R. & Sellmeyer, D & Todd, K & Sebastian, Anthony. (2001). Diet, evolution and aging--the pathophysiologic effects of the post-agricultural inversion of the potassium-to-sodium and base-to-chloride ratios in the human diet. *European journal of nutrition.* 40. 200-13.

160 Demigné C, Sabboh H, Rémésy C, Meneton P, (2004). Protective Effects of High Dietary Potassium: Nutritional and Metabolic Aspects. *The Journal of Nutrition.* Volume 134, Issue 11, November 2004, p. 2903–2906

161 Oberleithner H, Callies C, Kusche-Vihrog K, et al (2009). Potassium softens vascular endothelium and increases nitric oxide release. *PNAS* December 21.

162 Kovesdy CP, Appel LJ, Grams ME, Gutekunst L, McCullough PA, Palmer, BF, Pitt B, Sica DA, Townsend RR. (2017). Potassium Homeostasis in Health and Disease: A Scientific

Workshop Cosponsored by the National Kidney Foundation and the American Society of Hypertension. *Am J Kidney Dis. Special Report.* Elsevier Inc. Sun Y, Byon CH, Yang Y, Bradley WE, Dell'Italia LJ, Sanders PW, Agarwal A, Wu H, Chen Y,. (2017). Dietary potassium regulates vascular calcification and arterial stiffness. *JCI Insight.* 2017 Oct 5;2(19)

163   Lanfranco D'Elia, Gianvincenzo Barba, Francesco P. Cappuccio, Pasquale Strazzullo. (2011. Potassium Intake, Stroke, and Cardiovascular Disease. *J Am Coll Cardiol.* Mar, 57 (10) 1210-1219

164   Blanch N, Clifton PM, Petersen KS, Willoughby SR, Keogh JB. (2014). Effect of high potassium diet on endothelial function. *Nutrition, Metabolism & Cardiovascular Diseases.* 24, 983-989.

165   Blanch N, Clifton PM, Keogh JB. (2014). Postprandial effects of potassium supplementation on vascular function and blood pressure: a randomized cross-over study. *Nutrition, Metabolism & Cardiovascular Diseases.* 24, 148-154.

166   Jensen M.B., Lawaetz J.G., Andersson AM. (2016). Vitamin D deficiency and low ionized calcium are linked with semen quality and sex steroid levels in infertile men. *Human Reproduction,* Vol 31, Issue 8, Aug. p. 1875–1885

167   Dullo, P., & Vedi, N. (2008). Changes in serum calcium, magnesium and inorganic phosphorus levels during different phases of the menstrual cycle. *Journal of human reproductive sciences,* 1(2), 77–80.

168   Kim, K., Wactawski-Wende, J., Michels, K. A., Schliep, K. C., Plowden, T. C., Chaljub, E. N., & Mumford, S. L. (2018). Dietary minerals, reproductive hormone levels and sporadic anovulation: associations in healthy women with regular menstrual cycles. *The British journal of nutrition,* 120(1), 81–89. https://doi.org/10.1017/S0007114518000818

169   Kello D.M.V., Dekanić D., Kostial K. (1979) Influence of Sex and Dietary Calcium on Intestinal Cadmium Absorption in Rats, *Archives of Environmental Health: An International Journal,* 34:1, 30-33

170   Vitale, S. G., Caruso, S., Rapisarda, A., Cianci, S., & Cianci, A. (2018). Isoflavones, calcium, vitamin D and inulin improve quality of life, sexual function, body composition and metabolic parameters in menopausal women: result from a prospective, randomized, placebo-controlled, parallel-group study. Przeglad menopauzalny = *Menopause review,* 17(1), 32–38.

171   Bolland, M. J., Grey, A., Avenell, A., Gamble, G. D., & Reid, I. R. (2011). Calcium supplements with or without vitamin D and risk of cardiovascular events: reanalysis of the Women's Health Initiative limited access dataset and meta-analysis. *BMJ* (Clinical research ed.), 342, d2040.

172   Volpe S. L. (2013). Magnesium in disease prevention and overall health. *Advances in nutrition* (Bethesda, Md.), 4(3), 378S–83S.

173   Gröber, U., Schmidt, J., & Kisters, K. (2015). Magnesium in Prevention and Therapy. *Nutrients,* 7(9), 8199–8226.

174   Ma J1, Folsom AR, Melnick SL, Eckfeldt JH, Sharrett AR, Nabulsi AA, Hutchinson RG, Metcalf PA. (1995). Associations of serum and dietary magnesium with cardiovascular disease, hypertension, diabetes, insulin, and carotid arterial wall thickness: the ARIC study. Atherosclerosis Risk in Communities Study. *J Clin Epidemiol.* Jul;48(7):927-40.

175   Cahill, F., Shahidi, M., Shea, J., Wadden, D., Gulliver, W., Randell, E., ... Sun, G. (2013). High dietary magnesium intake is associated with low insulin resistance in the Newfoundland population. *PloS one,* 8(3), e58278. doi:10.1371/journal.pone.0058278

176   Moctezuma-Velázquez C1, Gómez-Sámano MÁ2, Cajas-Sánchez MB3, Reyes-Molina DL3, Galindo-Guzmán M1, Meza-Arana CE1, Cuevas-Ramos D2, Gómez-Pérez FJ2,

Gulias-Herrero A1.(2017). High Dietary Magnesium Intake is Significantly and Independently Associated with Higher Insulin Sensitivity in a Mexican-Mestizo Population: A Brief Cross-Sectional Report. *Rev Invest Clin.* 2017 Jan-Feb;69(1):40-46.

177 Cahill F1, Shahidi M, Shea J, Wadden D, Gulliver W, Randell E, Vasdev S, Sun G. (2013). High dietary magnesium intake is associated with low insulin resistance in the Newfoundland population. *PLoS One.* 2013;8(3):e58278. doi: 10.1371/journal.pone.0058278. Kumar P, Bhargava S, Agarwal PK, Garg A, Khosla A. (2019). Association of serum magnesium with type 2 diabetes mellitus and diabetic retinopathy. *J Family Med Prim Care.* 2019 May;8(5):1671-1677

178 Kirkland, A. E., Sarlo, G. L., & Holton, K. F. (2018). The Role of Magnesium in Neurological Disorders. *Nutrients,* 10(6), 730.

179 Maggio, M., De Vita, F., Lauretani, F., Nouvenne, A., Meschi, T., Ticinesi, A., Dominguez, L. J., Barbagallo, M., Dall'aglio, E., & Ceda, G. P. (2014). The Interplay between Magnesium and Testosterone in Modulating Physical Function in Men. *International journal of endocrinology,* 2014, 525249.

180 Chandra AK, Sengupta P, Goswami H, Sarkar M. (2013). Effects of dietary magnesium on testicular histology, steroidogenesis, spermatogenesis and oxidative stress markers in adult rats. *Indian J Exp Biol.*Jan;51(1):37-47.

181 Milton K. (1999). Nutritional characteristics of wild primate foods: do the diets of our closest living relatives have lessons for us? *Nutrition.* 1999 Jun;15(6):488-98.

182 Ronette R. Briefel, Karil Bialostosky, Jocelyn Kennedy-Stephenson, Margaret A. McDowell, R. Bethene Ervin, Jacqueline D. Wright, Zinc Intake of the U.S. Population: Findings from the Third National Health and Nutrition Examination Survey, 1988–1994, *The Journal of Nutrition,* Volume 130, Issue 5, May 2000, Pages 1367S–1373

183 Prasad, A.S., Mantzoros, C.S., Beck, F.W., Hess, J.W., & Brewer, G.J. (1996). Zinc status and serum testosterone levels of healthy adults. *Nutrition,* 12 5, 344-8 .

184 Prasad A. S. (2014). Zinc is an Antioxidant and Anti-Inflammatory Agent: Its Role in Human Health. *Frontiers in nutrition,* 1, 14.

185 Chu, A., Foster, M., & Samman, S. (2016). Zinc Status and Risk of Cardiovascular Diseases and Type 2 Diabetes Mellitus-A Systematic Review of Prospective Cohort Studies. *Nutrients,* 8(11), 707.

186 Chasapis CT, Loutsidou AC, Spiliopoulou CA, Stefanidou ME. (2012). Zinc and human health: an update. *Arch Toxicol.* 2012 Apr; 86(4):521-34.

187 Little PJ, Bhattacharya R, Moreyra AE, Korichneva IL. (2010). Zinc and cardiovascular disease. *Nutrition.* 2010 Nov-Dec; 26(11-12):1050-7.

188 Jarosz, M., Olbert, M., Wyszogrodzka, G., Młyniec, K., & Librowski, T. (2017). Antioxidant and anti-inflammatory effects of zinc. Zinc-dependent NF-κB signaling. *Inflammopharmacology,* 25(1), 11–24.

189 Omu, A. E., Al-Azemi, M. K., Al-Maghrebi, M., Mathew, C. T., Omu, F. E., Kehinde, E. O., Anim, J. T., Oriowo, M. A., & Memon, A. (2015). Molecular basis for the effects of zinc deficiency on spermatogenesis: An experimental study in the Sprague-dawley rat model. *Indian journal of urology* : IJU : journal of the Urological Society of India, 31(1), 57–64.

190 Dissanayake, D., Wijesinghe, P. S., Ratnasooriya, W. D., & Wimalasena, S. (2009). Effects of zinc supplementation on sexual behavior of male rats. *Journal of human reproductive sciences,* 2(2), 57–61.

191 Kim, K., Wactawski-Wende, J., Michels, K. A., Schliep, K. C., Plowden, T. C., Chaljub, E. N., & Mumford, S. L. (2018). Dietary minerals, reproductive hormone levels and sporadic anovulation: associations in healthy women with regular menstrual cycles. *The British journal of nutrition,* 120(1), 81–89.

192   Kurdoglu Z, Kurdoglu M, Demir H, Sahin HG. (2012). Serum trace elements and heavy metals in polycystic ovary syndrome. *Hum Exp Toxicol.* 2012;31(5):452-456.

193   Plasma selenium and plasma and erythrocyte glutathione peroxidase activity increase with estrogen during the menstrual cycle. Ha EJ, Smith AM *J Am Coll Nutr.* 2003 Feb; 22(1):43-51.

194   Pizzorno L. (2015). Nothing Boring About Boron. Integrative medicine (Encinitas, Calif.), 14(4), 35–48.

195   Studies on the bioavailability of zinc in humans: effects of heme and nonheme iron on the absorption of zinc.(1981).Solomons NW, Jacob RA. *Am J Clin Nutr.* 1981 Apr; 34(4):475-82.

196   Li, T. Y., Brennan, A. M., Wedick, N. M., Mantzoros, C., Rifai, N., & Hu, F. B. (2009). Regular consumption of nuts is associated with a lower risk of cardiovascular disease in women with type 2 diabetes. *The Journal of nutrition,* 139(7), 1333–1338.

197   Aune, D., Keum, N., Giovannucci, E., Fadnes, L. T., Boffetta, P., Greenwood, D. C., Tonstad, S., Vatten, L. J., Riboli, E., & Norat, T. (2016). Nut consumption and risk of cardiovascular disease, total cancer, all-cause and cause-specific mortality: a systematic review and dose-response meta-analysis of prospective studies. *BMC medicine, 14*(1), 207.

198   Coates, A., Hill, A. & Tan, S. (2018). Nuts and Cardiovascular Disease Prevention. *Curr Atheroscler Rep* 20, 48 (2018)

199   Salas-Huetos, A., Muralidharan, J., Galiè, S.,et al. (2019). Effect of Nut Consumption on Erectile and Sexual Function in Healthy Males: A Secondary Outcome Analysis of the FERTINUTS Randomized Controlled Trial. *Nutrients,* 11(6), 1372.

200   Aldemir, M., Okulu, E., Neşelioğlu, S. et al. (2011). Pistachio diet improves erectile function parameters and serum lipid profiles in patients with erectile dysfunction. *Int J Impot Res* 23, 32–38 (2011)

201   Negrişanu G, Roşu M, Bolte B, Lefter D, Dabelea D. (1999). Effects of 3-month treatment with the antioxidant alpha-lipoic acid in diabetic peripheral neuropathy. *Rom J Intern Med.* Jul-Sep;37(3):297-306.

202   Ros E. (2009). Nuts and novel biomarkers of cardiovascular disease, *The American Journal of Clinical Nutrition,* Volume 89, Issue 5. Pages 1649S–1656S

203   Cortés B, Núñez I, Cofán M, et al (2006). Acute Effects of High-Fat Meals Enriched With Walnuts or Olive Oil on Postprandial Endothelial Function. *Journal of the American College of Cardiology* Volume 48, Issue 8, Pages 1666-1671

204   McDonagh STJ1, Wylie LJ1, Thompson C1, Vanhatalo A1, Jones AM1. (2019). Potential benefits of dietary nitrate ingestion in healthy and clinical populations: A brief review. *Eur J Sport Sci.* Feb;19(1):15-29 Murphy M, Eliot K, Heuertz R, Weiss E. (2012). Whole Beetroot Consumption Acutely Improves Running Performance. *Journal of the American Academy of Nutrition and Dietetics.* 112(4):548-52 · April

205   Liu AH1, Bondonno CP, Croft KD, Puddey IB, Woodman RJ, Rich L, Ward NC, Vita JA, Hodgson JM. (2013). Effects of a nitrate-rich meal on arterial stiffness and blood pressure in healthy volunteers. *Nitric Oxide* Volume 35, 30 November 2013, Pages 123-130

206   Hord NG, Tang Y, Bryan NS. (2009). Food sources of nitrates and nitrites: the physiologic context for potential health benefits. *The American Journal of Clinical Nutrition.* Volume 90, Issue 1, July 2009, Pages 1–10

Ancient Chinese Wisdom for Great Sex

207   Van Gulik R. (1961). Sexual Life in Ancient China: A Preliminary Survey of Chinese Sex and Society from ca. 1500 B. C. till 1644 A. D. Sterling Publishing. New York.

208 Goldin PR. (2001). *The Culture of Sex in Ancient China.* University of Hawaii Press. Honolulu.

209 Radford L. (n.d.) *What Sex Was Like in Pre-Modern China.* Retrieved from: https://www.ranker.com/list/in-ancient-china/lyra-radford

210 Maciocia G. *Sexual Life in Chinese Medicine.* Giovanni Maciocia. Retrieved 7/10/20 from https://giovanni-maciocia.com/sexual-life-in-chinese-medicine/

211 Wiseman N., Ellis A. (1996). *Fundamentals of Chinese Medicine.* Paradigm Publications. Brookline, Massachusetts.

Traditional Chinese Dietetics

212 Kastner J. (2009). *Chinese Nutrition Therapy Dietetics in Traditional Chinese Medicine (TCM).* Thieme, New York.

213 Maoshing N., McNease C. (2009). *The Tao of Nutrition.* Tao of Wellness Press. Los Angeles.

Great Sex is in the Living and Breathing

214 Lamina, S., Agbanusi, E., & Nwacha, R. C. (2011). Effects of aerobic exercise in the management of erectile dysfunction: a meta analysis study on randomized controlled trials. *Ethiopian journal of health, sciences* 21(3), 195–201.

215 Jiannine L. M. (2018). An investigation of the relationship between physical fitness, self-concept, and sexual functioning. *Journal of education and health promotion,* 7, 57.

216 White JR, Case DA, McWhirter D, Mattison AM. (1990). Enhanced sexual behavior in exercising men. *Arch Sex Behav.* 1990;19(3):193-209.

217 Hsiao W, Shrewsberry AB, Moses KA, et al. (2012). Exercise is associated with better erectile function in men under 40 as evaluated by the International Index of Erectile Function. *J Sex Med.* 2012;9(2):524-530

218 Gerbild, H., Larsen, C. M., Graugaard, C., & Areskoug Joséfsson, K. (2018). Physical Activity to Improve Erectile Function: A Systematic Review of Intervention Studies. *Sexual medicine,* 6(2), 75–89.

219 Fergus KB, Gaither TW, Baradaran N, Glidden DV, Cohen AJ, Breyer BN. (2019). Exercise Improves Self-Reported Sexual Function Among Physically Active Adults. *J Sex Med.* 2019;16(8):1236-1245.

220 Meston CM, Gorzalka BB. (1996). The effects of immediate, delayed, and residual sympathetic activation on sexual arousal in women. *Behav Res Ther.* 1996 Feb; 34(2):143-8.

221 Petriz, B.A., Castro, A.P., Almeida, J.A. et al. (2014). Exercise induction of gut microbiota modifications in obese, non-obese and hypertensive rats. *BMC Genomics* 15, 511

222 Golbidi, Saeid & Daiber, Andreas & Korac, Bato & Li, Huige & Essop, M Faadiel & Laher, Ismail. (2017). Health Benefits of Fasting and Caloric Restriction. *Current Diabetes Reports.* 17. 10.1007/s11892-017-0951-7.

223 Silverstein RG, Brown AC, Roth HD, Britton WB. (2011). Effects of mindfulness training on body awareness to sexual stimuli: implications for female sexual dysfunction. *Psychosom Med.* 2011 Nov-Dec; 73(9):817-25.

224 Alsubiheen A, Petrofsky J, Daher N, Lohman E, Balbas E, Lee H. (2017). Tai Chi with mental imagery theory improves soleus H-reflex and nerve conduction velocity in patients with type 2 diabetes. *Complement Ther Med.* 2017;31:59-64.

225 Gupta R, Verma M, Gupta R, Gupta S, Anand KS. (2010). Yoga in female sexual functions. Dhikav V, Karmarkar G, *J Sex Med.* 2010 Feb; 7(2 Pt 2):964-70.

Heavy Metal Exposure

226 Kim JJ., Kim YS., Kumar V. (2019).Heavy metal toxicity: An update of chelating thera-peutic strategies. *J Trace Elem Med Biol.* 2019 Jul;54:226-231.

227 Pawankar R, Canonica GW, Holgate ST, Lockey RF, editors. *WAO White book on Allergy* 2011–2012 [Internet]. Milwaukee, WI (US): World Allergy Organization, 2013:228.

228 Rana SV. (2014). Perspectives in endocrine toxicity of heavy metals--a review. *Biol Trace Elem Res.* 2014 Jul;160(1):1-14.

229 Otto Hänninen, Anne B. Knol, Matti Jantunen, Tek-Ang Lim, André Conrad, Marianne Rappolder, Paolo Carrer, Anna-Clara Fanetti, Rokho Kim, Jurgen Buekers, Rudi Torfs, Ivano Iavarone, Thomas Classen, Claudia Hornberg, Odile C.L. Mekel, and the EBoDE Working Group.(2014).Environmental Burden of Disease in Europe: Assessing Nine Risk Factors in Six Countries. *Environmental Health Perspectives.* 122:5

230 Dotse, CK. (2010). "Assessing Commercial Organic and Conventionally Grown Vegeta-bles by Monitoring Selected Heavy Metals Found in Them." (2010). *Electronic Theses and Dissertations.* Paper 1715. https://dc.etsu.edu/etd/1715

231 Flanagan PR, Chamberlain MJ, Valberg LS. (1982). The relationship between iron and lead absorption in humans. *Am J Clin Nutr.* 1982 Nov;36(5):823-9.

232 Jackson, L. W., Howards, P. P., Wactawski-Wende, J., & Schisterman, E. F. (2011). The association between cadmium, lead and mercury blood levels and reproductive hormones among healthy, premenopausal women. *Human reproduction* (Oxford, England), 26(10), 2887–2895.

233 Betts K. S. (2010). Do metals meddle with puberty in girls? Lead, cadmium, and altered hormone levels. *Environmental health perspectives,* 118(12), a542.

234 Pollack, A. Z., Schisterman, E. F., Goldman, L. R., Mumford, S. L., Albert, P. S., Jones, R. L., & Wactawski-Wende, J. (2011). Cadmium, lead, and mercury in relation to reproduc-tive hormones and anovulation in premenopausal women. *Environmental health perspec-tives,* 119(8), 1156–1161.

235 Ng TB, Liu WK.(1990).Toxic effect of heavy metals on cells isolated from the rat adrenal and testis. *In Vitro Cell Dev Biol.* 1990 Jan;26(1):24-8.

236 Wiebe JP, Barr KJ, Buckingham KDEffect of prenatal and neonatal exposure to lead on gonadotropin receptors and steroidogenesis in rat ovaries. *J Toxicol Environ Health.* 1988; 24(4):461-76. Nampoothiri LP, Gupta S (2006). Simultaneous effect of lead and cadmium on granulosa cells: a cellular model for ovarian toxicity. *Reprod Toxicol.* 2006 Feb; 21(2):179-85.

237 Junaid M, Chowdhuri DK, Narayan R, Shanker R, Saxena DK. (1997). Lead-induced changes in ovarian follicular development and maturation in mice. *J Toxicol Environ Health.* 1997 Jan; 50(1):31-40.

238 Brama M, Gnessi L, Basciani S, Cerulli N, Politi L, Spera G, Mariani S, Cherubini S, Scotto d'Abusco A, Scandurra R, Migliaccio S. (2007). Cadmium induces mitogenic signaling in breast cancer cell by an ERalpha-dependent mechanism. *Mol Cell Endocrinol.* 2007 Jan 29; 264(1-2):102-8

239 Martin MB, Reiter R, Pham T, Avellanet YR, Camara J, Lahm M, Pentecost E, Pratap K, Gilmore BA, Divekar S, Dagata RS, Bull JL, Stoica A. (2002). Estrogen-like activity of metals in MCF-7 breast cancer cells. *Endocrinology.* 2003 Jun; 144(6):2425-36.

240 Jackson LW, Zullo MD, Goldberg JM. (2008). The association between heavy metals, endometriosis and uterine myomas among premenopausal women: *National Health and Nutrition Examination Survey* 1999-2002. *Hum Reprod.* 2008 Mar; 23(3):679-87.

241   Chang SH, Cheng BH, Lee SL, Chuang HY, Yang CY, Sung FC, Wu TN. (2006). Low blood lead concentration in association with infertility in women. *Environ Res.* 2006 Jul; 101(3):380-6.

242   Jackson, L. W., Howards, P. P., Wactawski-Wende, J., & Schisterman, E. F. (2011). The association between cadmium, lead and mercury blood levels and reproductive hormones among healthy, premenopausal women. *Human reproduction* (Oxford, England), 26(10), 2887–2895.

243   Soliman, A., De Sanctis, V., & Elalaily, R. (2014). Nutrition and pubertal development. *Indian journal of endocrinology and metabolism,* 18(Suppl 1), S39–S47.

244   Staff, N. P., & Windebank, A. J. (2014). Peripheral neuropathy due to vitamin deficiency, toxins, and medications. *Continuum* (Minneapolis, Minn.), 20(5 Peripheral Nervous System Disorders), 1293–1306.

245   Hallanger IG1, Jørgensen EH, Fuglei E, Ahlstrøm Ø, Muir DC, Jenssen BM.(2012). Dietary contaminant exposure affects plasma testosterone, but not thyroid hormones, vitamin A, and vitamin E, in male juvenile arctic foxes (Vulpes lagopus). *J Toxicol Environ Health A.* 2012;75(21):1298-313.

246   Grennan AK. (2011). Metallothioneins, a Diverse Protein Family. *Plant Physiology* Apr 2011, 155 (4) 1750-1751

247   Ruttkay-Nedecky, B., Nejdl, L., Gumulec, J., Zitka, O., Masarik, M., Eckschlager, T., Stiborova, M., Adam, V., & Kizek, R. (2013). The role of metallothionein in oxidative stress. *International journal of molecular sciences,* 14(3), 6044–6066.

248   Suresh Kumar K, Dahms HU, Won EJ, Lee JS, Shin KH. (2015). Microalgae - A promising tool for heavy metal remediation. *Ecotoxicol Environ Saf.* 2015 Mar;113:329-52.

249   Adams, J., Howsmon, D. P., Kruger, U., Geis, E., Gehn, E., Fimbres, V., Pollard, E., Mitchell, J., Ingram, J., Hellmers, R., Quig, D., & Hahn, J. (2017). Significant Association of Urinary Toxic Metals and Autism-Related Symptoms-A Nonlinear Statistical Analysis with Cross Validation. *PloS one,* 12(1).

250   Walker SJ., Segal J, Aschner M. (2006) Cultured lymphocytes from autistic children and non-autistic siblings up-regulate heat shock protein RNA in response to thimerosal challenge, *Neuro Toxicology,* Volume 27, Issue 5, 2006,Pages 685-692.

251   Flora SJS., Mittal M., Mehta A. (2008). Heavy metal induced oxidative stress & its possible reversal by chelation therapy. *Indian J Med Res* 128, October 2008, pp 501-523

252   Sears M. E. (2013). Chelation: harnessing and enhancing heavy metal detoxification--a review. *The Scientific World Journal,* 2013, 219840. https://doi.org/10.1155/2013/219840

253   Greger M, (2017). Best Foods for Lead Poisoning: Chlorella, Cilantro, Tomatoes, Moringa? M.D. *FACLM* May 31st, 2017 Volume 36 https://nutritionfacts.org/video/best-foods-for-lead-poisoning-chlorella-cilantro-tomatoes-moringa/

254   Sears M. E. (2013). Chelation: harnessing and enhancing heavy metal detoxification--a review. *The Scientific World Journal,* 2013, 219840. https://doi.org/10.1155/2013/219840

255   Berglund, M., Akesson, A., Nermell, B., & Vahter, M. (1994). Intestinal absorption of dietary cadmium in women depends on body iron stores and fiber intake. *Environmental health perspectives,* 102(12), 1058–1066.

256   Zhai, Q., Narbad, A., & Chen, W. (2015). Dietary strategies for the treatment of cadmium and lead toxicity. *Nutrients,* 7(1), 552–571.

257   Abdalla FH1, Bellé LP, De Bona KS, Bitencourt PE, Pigatto AS, Moretto MB. (2009). Allium sativum L. extract prevents methyl mercury-induced cytotoxicity in peripheral blood leukocytes (LS).*Food Chem Toxicol.* 2010 Jan;48(1):417-21. doi: 10.1016/j.fct.2009.10.033. Epub 2009 Oct 29.

258   Zhai, Q., Narbad, A., & Chen, W. (2015). Dietary strategies for the treatment of cadmium and lead toxicity. *Nutrients,* 7(1), 552–571.

259   Uchikawa T, Kumamoto Y, Maruyama I, Kumamoto S, Ando Y, Yasutake A.Enhanced elimination of tissue methylmercury in Parachlorella beijerinckii-fed mice. *J Toxicol Sci.* 2011 Jan;36(1):121-6.

260   Nwokocha CR1, Nwokocha MI, Aneto I, Obi J, Udekweleze DC, Olatunde B, Owu DU, Iwuala MO. (2012). Comparative analysis on the effect of Lycopersicon esculentum (tomato) in reducing cadmium, mercury and lead accumulation in liver. *Food Chem Toxicol.* 2012 Jun;50(6):2070-3.

261   James HM, Hilburn ME, Blair JA.Effects of meals and meal times on uptake of lead from the gastrointestinal tract in humans.*Hum Toxicol.* 1985 Jul;4(4):401-7.

262   Senapati SK1, Dey S, Dwivedi SK, Swarup D. (2001). Effect of garlic (Allium sativum L.) extract on tissue lead level in rats.J Ethnopharmacol. 2001 Aug;76(3):229-32.

263   Kianoush S1, Balali-Mood M, Mousavi SR, Moradi V, Sadeghi M, Dadpour B, Rajabi O, Shakeri MT. (2012). Comparison of therapeutic effects of garlic and d-Penicillamine in patients with chronic occupational lead poisoning. *Basic Clin Pharmacol Toxicol.* 2012 May;110(5):476-81. doi: 10.1111/j.1742-7843.2011.00841.x. Epub 2011 Dec 29.

264   Mustafa HN. (2015). Potential Alleviation of Chlorella Vulgaris and Zingiber officinale on Lead-Induced Testicular Toxicity: an Ultrastructural Study. *Folia Biol* (Krakow). 2015;63(4):269-78.

265   Sharma V1, Kansal L, Sharma A. (2010).Prophylactic efficacy of Coriandrum sativum (Coriander) on testis of lead-exposed mice. *Biol Trace Elem Res.* 2010 Sep;136(3):337-54.

266   Sharma V1, Kansal L, Sharma A. (2010).Prophylactic efficacy of Coriandrum sativum (Coriander) on testis of lead-exposed mice. *Biol Trace Elem Res.* 2010 Sep;136(3):337-54.

267   Lakshmi BV, Sudhakar M, Aparna M. (2013). Protective potential of Black grapes against lead induced oxidative stress in rats. *Environ Toxicol Pharmacol.* 2013 May;35(3):361-8.

268   García-Niño WR1, Pedraza-Chaverrí J2. (2014). Protective effect of curcumin against heavy metals-induced liver damage.Food *Chem Toxicol.* 2014 Jul;69:182-201. doi: 10.1016/j.fct.2014.04.016. Epub 2014 Apr 18.

269   Biswas J1, Sinha D, Mukherjee S, Roy S, Siddiqi M, Roy M. (2010). Curcumin protects DNA damage in a chronically arsenic-exposed population of West Bengal. *Hum Exp Toxicol.* 2010 Jun;29(6):513-24. doi: 10.1177/0960327109359020. Epub 2010 Jan 7.

Electromagnietic Fields

270   Sears M. E. (2013). Chelation: harnessing and enhancing heavy metal detoxification--a review. *The Scientific World Journal,* 2013, 219840.

271   Lai H, Singh NP. (2004). Magnetic-field-induced DNA strand breaks in brain cells of the rat. *Environ Health Perspect.* 2004 May; 112(6):687-94.

272   Havas Magda. (1976). Biological effects of electromagnetic radiation. *Engineering and Technology History.* (1976).

273   London SJ, Thomas DC, Bowman JD, Sobel E, Cheng TC, Peters JM. (1991). Exposure to residential electric and magnetic fields and risk of childhood leukemia. *Am J Epidemiol.* 1991 Nov 1; 134(9):923-37.

274   Sobel E, Dunn M, Davanipour Z, Qian Z, Chui HC. (1996). Elevated risk of Alzheimer's disease among workers with likely electromagnetic field exposure. *Neurology.* 1996;47(6):1477-1481.

275   Saili L, Hanini A, Smirani C, Azzouz I, Azzouz A, Sakly M, Abdelmelek H, Bouslama Z. (2015). Effects of acute exposure to WIFI signals (2.45GHz) on heart variability and blood pressure in Albinos rabbit. *Environ Toxicol Pharmacol.* 2015 Sep; 40(2):600-5.

276   A. Agarwal, F. Deepinder, R.K. Sharma, G. Ranga, J. Li. (2008). Effect of cell phone usage on semen analysis in men attending infertility clinic: an observational study. *Fertil Steril,* 89 (2008), pp. 124-128

277   Hardell L, & Carlberg M, Gee D. (2015). Mobile phone use and brain tumour risk: early warnings, early actions? In *Late lessons from early warnings: science, precaution, innovation. European Environment Agency* 509-529.

278   Sistani S, Fatemi I, Shafeie SA, Kaeidi A, Azin M, Shamsizadeh A. (2019).The effect of Wi-Fi electromagnetic waves on neuronal response properties in rat barrel cortex. *Somatosens Mot Res.* 2019;36(4):292-297.

279   Panagopoulos DJ, Johansson O, Carlo GL. (2015). Polarization: A Key Difference between Man-made and Natural Electromagnetic Fields, in regard to Biological Activity. *Sci Rep.* 2015 Oct 12; 5():14914.

280   Morgan LL, Miller AB, Sasco A, Davis DL. (2015). Mobile phone radiation causes brain tumors and should be classified as a probable human carcinogen (2A) (review). *Int J Oncol.* 2015;46(5):1865-1871.

281   Hardell L, & Carlberg M, Gee D. (2015). Mobile phone use and brain tumour risk: early warnings, early actions? In Late lessons from early warnings: science, precaution, innovation. *European Environment Agency* p. 515.

282   Leszczynski D, Joenväärä S, Reivinen J, Kuokka R. (2002). Non-thermal activation of the hsp27/p38MAPK stress pathway by mobile phone radiation in human endothelial cells: molecular mechanism for cancer- and blood-brain barrier-related effects. *Differentiation.* 2002;70(2-3):120-129.

283   Volkow ND, Tomasi D, Wang GJ, et al. (2011). Effects of cell phone radiofrequency signal exposure on brain glucose metabolism. *JAMA.* 2011;305(8):808-813.

284   Obajuluwa, A. O., Akinyemi, A. J., Afolabi, O. B., Adekoya, K., Sanya, J. O., & Ishola, A. O. (2017). Exposure to radio-frequency electromagnetic waves alters acetylcholinesterase gene expression, exploratory and motor coordination-linked behaviour in male rats. *Toxicology reports,* 4, 530–534.

285   Vesselinova L. (2015). Body mass index as a risk prediction and prevention factor for professional mixed low-intensity EMF burden. *Electromagn Biol Med.* 2015;34(3):238-243.

286   Asghari, A., Khaki, A. A., Rajabzadeh, A., & Khaki, A. (2016). A review on Electromagnetic fields (EMFs) and the reproductive system. *Electronic physician,* 8(7), 2655–2662.

287   Singh, R., Nath, R., Mathur, A. K., & Sharma, R. S. (2018). Effect of radiofrequency radiation on reproductive health. *The Indian journal of medical research,* 148(Suppl), S92–S99. https://doi.org/10.4103/ijmr.IJMR_1056_18

288   Gye MC, Park CJ. (2012). Effect of electromagnetic field exposure on the reproductive system. *Clin Exp Reprod Med.* 2012 Mar; 39(1):1-9.

289   I. Fejes, Z. Závaczki, J. Szöllosi, S. Koloszár, J. Daru, L. Kovács, et al.(2005). Is there a relationship between cell phone use and semen quality? *Arch Androl,* 51 (2005), pp. 385-393

290   Yildirim ME., Kaynar M., Huseyin B. et al. (2015). What is harmful for male fertility: Cell phone or the wireless internet? *The Kaohsiung Journal of Medical Sciences.* Volume 31, Issue 9, September 2015, Pages 480-484

291   Kim YW, Kim HS, Lee JS, Kim YJ, Lee SK, Seo JN, Jung KC, Kim N, Gimm YM. (2009). Effects of 60 Hz 14 microT magnetic field on the apoptosis of testicular germ cell in mice. *Bioelectromagnetics.* 2009 Jan; 30(1):66-72.

292   A. Agarwal, F. Deepinder, R.K. Sharma, G. Ranga, J. Li. (2008). Effect of cell phone usage on semen analysis in men attending infertility clinic: an observational study. *Fertil Steril,* 89 (2008), pp. 124-128

293   Iorio R, Scrimaglio R, Rantucci E, Delle Monache S, Di Gaetano A, Finetti N, Francavilla F, Santucci R, Tettamanti E, Colonna R. (2007). A preliminary study of oscillating electromagnetic field effects on human spermatozoon motility. *Bioelectromagnetics.* 2007 Jan; 28(1):72-5.

294   Shokri S, Soltani A, Kazemi M, Sardari D, Mofrad FB. (2015). Effects of Wi-Fi (2.45 GHz) Exposure on Apoptosis, Sperm Parameters and Testicular Histomorphometry in Rats: A Time Course Study. *Cell J.* 2015 Summer; 17(2):322-31.

295   Houston BJ, Nixon B, King BV, De Iuliis GN, Aitken RJ. (2016). The effects of radiofrequency electromagnetic radiation on sperm function. *Reproduction.* 2016;152(6):R263-R276.

296   Asghari, A., Khaki, A. A., Rajabzadeh, A., & Khaki, A. (2016). A review on Electromagnetic fields (EMFs) and the reproductive system. *Electronic physician,* 8(7), 2655–2662.

297   Burchard JF, Nguyen DH, Block E. (1998). Progesterone concentrations during estrous cycle of dairy cows exposed to electric and magnetic fields. *Bioelectromagnetics.* 1998; 19(7):438-43.

298   Roshangar L, Hamdi BA, Khaki AA, Rad JS. (2014). Effect of low-frequency electromagnetic field exposure on oocyte differentiation and follicular development. Soleimani-Rad S. *Adv Biomed Res.* 2014; 3():76.

299   Nelson JF, Karelus K, Bergman MD, Felicio LS. (1995). Neuroendocrine involvement in aging: evidence from studies of reproductive aging and caloric restriction. *Neurobiol Aging.* 1995 Sep-Oct; 16(5):837-43; discussion 855-6.

300   Saygin M, Ozmen O, Erol O, Ellidag HY, Ilhan I, Aslankoc R. (2018). The impact of electromagnetic radiation (2.45 GHz, Wi-Fi) on the female reproductive system: The role of vitamin C. *Toxicol Ind Health.* 2018;34(9):620-630.

301   Jung KA, Ahn HS, Lee YS, Gye MC. (2007). Effect of a 20 kHz sawtooth magnetic field exposure on the estrous cycle in mice. *J Microbiol Biotechnol.* 2007 Mar; 17(3):398-402.

302   Khaki A, Ranjbar M, Rahimi F, Ghahramanian A. (2011). The effects of electromagnetic field (EMFs) on ovary in rat. *Ultrasound in obstetrics and gynecology.* 2011;38:269.

303   Cecconi S, Gualtieri G, Di Bartolomeo A, Troiani G, Cifone MG, Canipari R. (2000). Evaluation of the effects of extremely low frequency electromagnetic fields on mammalian follicle development. *Hum Reprod.* 2000 Nov; 15(11):2319-25.

304   Asghari, A., Khaki, A. A., Rajabzadeh, A., & Khaki, A. (2016). A review on Electromagnetic fields (EMFs) and the reproductive system. *Electronic physician,* 8(7), 2655–2662.

305   Cao YN, Zhang Y, Liu Y. (2006). Effects of exposure to extremely low frequency electromagnetic fields on reproduction of female mice and development of offsprings]. *Zhonghua Lao Dong Wei Sheng Zhi Ye Bing Za Zhi.* 2006 Aug; 24(8):468-70.

306   Süleyman Daşdag', M. Zülküf Akdag', Orhan Ayyıldız, Ömer C. Demirtaş, Murat Yayla & Cemil Sert (2000). DO CELLULAR PHONES ALTER BLOOD PARAMETERS AND BIRTH WEIGHT OF RATS?, Electro- and *Magnetobiology,* 19:1, 107-113

307   Borhani N, Rajaei F, Salehi Z, Javadi A. (2011). Analysis of DNA fragmentation in mouse embryos exposed to an extremely low-frequency electromagnetic field. *Electromagn Biol Med.* 2011;30(4):246-252

308   Goldhaber MK, Polen MR, Hiatt RA. (1988). The risk of miscarriage and birth defects among women who use visual display terminals during pregnancy. *Am J Ind Med.* 1988; 13(6):695-706.

309   Gye MC, Park CJ. (2012). Effect of electromagnetic field exposure on the reproductive system. *Clin Exp Reprod Med.* 2012 Mar; 39(1):1-9.

310   Belyaev I., Dean A., Eger H., Hubmann G. (2016). EUROPAEM EMF Guideline 2016 for the prevention, diagnosis and treatment of EMF-related health problems and illnesses. *Reviews on environmental health.* 31. 10.1515/reveh-2016-0011.

311 Volkov A.G., Markin V.S. (2015) Active and Passive Electrical Signaling in Plants. In: Lüttge U., Beyschlag W. (eds) Progress in Botany. *Progress in Botany (Genetics - Physiology - Systematics - Ecology)*, vol 76. Springer, Cham

312 Corsini E., Acosta V., Baddour N., et al. (2011). Search for plant biomagnetism with a sensitive atomic magnetometer. *Journal of Applied Physics* 109:7

313 Oral B, Guney M, Ozguner F, Karahan N, Mungan T, Comlekci S, Cesur G. (2006). Endometrial apoptosis induced by a 900-MHz mobile phone: preventive effects of vitamins E and C. *Adv Ther.* 2006 Nov-Dec; 23(6):957-73.

314 Devrim E, Ergüder IB, Kılıçoğlu B, Yaykaşlı E, Cetin R, Durak I. (2008). Effects of Electromagnetic Radiation Use on Oxidant/Antioxidant Status and DNA Turn-over Enzyme Activities in Erythrocytes and Heart, Kidney, Liver, and Ovary Tissues From Rats: Possible Protective Role of Vitamin C. *Toxicol Mech Methods.* 2008;18(9):679-683.

315 Saygin M, Ozmen O, Erol O, Ellidag HY, Ilhan I, Aslankoc R. (2018). The impact of electromagnetic radiation (2.45 GHz, Wi-Fi) on the female reproductive system: The role of vitamin C. *Toxicol Ind Health.* 2018;34(9):620-630.

316 Bakhshaeshi M, Khaki A, Fathiazad F, Khaki AA, Ghadamkheir E. (2012). Anti-oxidative role of quercetin derived from Allium cepa on aldehyde oxidase (OX-LDL) and hepatocytes apoptosis in streptozotocin-induced diabetic rat. *Asian Pac J Trop Biomed.* 2012 Jul; 2(7):528-31.

317 Hemadi M, Saki G, Rajabzadeh A, Khodadadi A, Sarkaki A. (2013). The effects of honey and vitamin E administration on apoptosis in testes of rat exposed to noise stress. *J Hum Reprod Sci.* 2013 Jan; 6(1):54-8

318 Lewicka, Małgorzata & Zawadzka, Magdalena & Henrykowska, Gabriela & Rutkowski, Maciej & Pacholski, Krzysztof & Buczyński, Andrzej. (2017). Antioxidant response of vitamin A during the exposure of blood platelets to electromagnetic radiation generated by LCD monitors – in vitro study. *European Journal of Biological Research.* 10.5281/zenodo.321600

319 Asghari, A., Khaki, A. A., Rajabzadeh, A., & Khaki, A. (2016). A review on Electromagnetic fields (EMFs) and the reproductive system. *Electronic physician.* 8(7), 2655–2662.

Great Sex from Your Partner's Eyes

320 Bridges, Ana & Bergner, Raymond & Hesson-McInnis, Matthew. (2003). Romantic Partners Use of Pornography: Its Significance for Women. *Journal of sex & marital therapy.* 29. 1-14.

321 Chida Y, Steptoe A. (2009). The association of anger and hostility with future coronary heart disease: a meta-analytic review of prospective evidence. *J Am Coll Cardiol.* 2009;53(11):936-946. 8

Aphrodisiacs: Fluffers of the Gods

322 Gulland S. (2014, March) "Spanish Fly"—a deadly Viagra of the past. Sandra Gulland http://www.sandragulland.com/spanish-fly-a-deadly-viagra-of-the-past/

323 Quartz India. Ishq. (2017). The ancient Indian aphrodisiacs from the Kamasutra lurking in your cupboard. Retrieved online: https://qz.com/india/994082/the-ancient-indian-aphrodisiacs-from-the-kamasutra-lurking-in-your-cupboard/

324   Lampiao F, Krom D, du Plessis SS. (2008). The in vitro effects of Mondia whitei on human sperm motility parameters. Phytother Res. Sep; 22(9):1272-3.

325   Hellen A. Oketch-Rabah (2012) Mondia whitei, a Medicinal Plant from Africa with Aphrodisiac and Antidepressant Properties: A Review, Journal of Dietary Supplements, 9:4, 272-284

326   Oludele, O., Idris, B., Benard, O., Pius, U., & Olufunso, O. (2018). Mondia whitei, an African Spice Inhibits Mitochondrial Permeability Transition in Rat Liver. Preventive nutrition and food science, 23(3), 206–213.

327   Adebayo, A. A., Oboh, G., & Ademosun, A. O. (2019). Almond-supplemented diet improves sexual

328   Qureshi S, Shah A.H., M., Ageel T. and A.M. (1989). Studies on Herbal Aphrodisiacs Used in Arab System of Medicine. The American Journal of Chinese Medicine. Vol. 17, No. 01n02, pp. 57-63

329   Sutyarso, Kanedi, M., & Rosa, E. (2015). Effects of Black Pepper (Piper nigrum Linn.) Extract on Sexual Drive in Male Mice. Research Journal of Medicinal Plant, 9, 42-47.

330   Lee, J. S., Kim, S. G., Kim, H. K., Baek, S. Y., & Kim, C. M. (2012). Acute effects of capsaicin on proopioimelanocortin mRNA levels in the arcuate nucleus of Sprague-Dawley rats. Psychiatry investigation, 9(2), 187–190.

331   T Ilhan & H Erdost (2013) Effects of capsaicin on testis ghrelin expression in mice, Biotechnic & Histochemistry, 88:1, 10-18

332   McCarty, M. F., DiNicolantonio, J. J., & O'Keefe, J. H. (2015). Capsaicin may have important potential for promoting vascular and metabolic health. Open heart, 2(1), e000262.

333   Tang, X., Olatunji, O. J., Zhou, Y., & Hou, X. (2017). In vitro and in vivo aphrodisiac properties of the seed extract from Allium tuberosum on corpus cavernosum smooth muscle relaxation and sexual behavior parameters in male Wistar rats. BMC complementary and alternative medicine, 17(1), 510.

334   Parker G1, Parker I, Brotchie H. Mood state effects of chocolate. J Affect Disord. 2006 Jun;92(2-3):149-59. Epub 2006 Mar 20.

335   Tajuddin, Ahmad, S., Latif, A., & Qasmi, I. A. (2003). Aphrodisiac activity of 50% ethanolic extracts of Myristica fragrans Houtt. (nutmeg) and Syzygium aromaticum (L) Merr. & Perry. (clove) in male mice: a comparative study. BMC complementary and alternative medicine, 3, 6.

336   Raghav Kumar Mishra, Shio Kumar Singh. ((2008). Safety assessment of Syzygium aromaticum flower bud (clove) extract with respect to testicular function in mice. Food and Chemical Toxicology. Volume 46, Issue 10, 2008, Pages 3333-3338,

337   Abdu S. B. (2018). Ameliorative Influence of Ajwa Dates on Ochratoxin A-Induced Testis Toxicity. Journal of microscopy and ultrastructure, 6(3), 134–138. doi:10.4103/JMAU. JMAU_14_18

338   Michael HN1, Salib JY, Eskander EF. (2013). Bioactivity of diosmetin glycosides isolated from the epicarp of date fruits, Phoenix dactylifera, on the biochemical profile of alloxan diabetic male rats. Phytother Res. May;27(5):699-704

339   Saryono, Saryono & Dwi, Mekar & Rahmawati, Eni. (2018). EFFECTS OF DATES FRUIT (PHOENIX DACTYLIFERA L.) IN THE FEMALE REPRODUCTIVE PROCESS. Current Trends in Nutraceuticals. 03.

340   The Herb Society of America's Essential Guide to Dill. Retrieved Online: https://www. herbsociety.org/file_download/inline/0191822e-0527-4cac-afb6-99d2caab6b78

341   Iamsaard, S., Prabsattroo, T., Sukhorum, W., Muchimapura, S., Srisaard, P., Uabundit, N., Thukhammee, W., & Wattanathorn, J. (2013). Anethum graveolens Linn. (dill) extract

enhances the mounting frequency and level of testicular tyrosine protein phosphorylation in rats. *Journal of Zhejiang University. Science.* B, 14(3), 247–252.

342   Mahboubi M. (2019). Foeniculum vulgare as Valuable Plant in Management of Women's Health.*J Menopausal Med.* 2019 Apr;25(1):1-14.

343   Abedi, P., Najafian, M., Yaralizadeh, M., & Namjoyan, F. (2018). Effect of fennel vaginal cream on sexual function in postmenopausal women: A double blind randomized controlled trial. *Journal of medicine and life,* 11(1), 24–28.

344   Khadivzadeh, T., Najafi, M. N., Kargarfard, L., Ghazanfarpour, M., Dizavandi, F. R., & Khorsand, I. (2018). Effect of Fennel on the Health Status of Menopausal Women: A Systematic and Meta-analysis. *Journal of menopausal medicine,* 24(1), 67–74.

345   Asghari, A., Khaki, A. A., Rajabzadeh, A., & Khaki, A. (2016). A review on Electromagnetic fields (EMFs) and the reproductive system. *Electronic physician.* 8(7), 2655–2662.

346   The Herb Society of America Quick Facts on Fennel. Retrieved online: https://www.herbsociety.org/file_download/inline/520b142e-66f4-45dc-b151-59283956b21e

347   Garlic. An Herb Society of America Guide. Retrieved online: https://www.herbsociety.org/file_download/inline/f751abad-cc5c-414f-89a5-b9e6b012ea70

348   al-Bekairi AM1, Shah AH, Qureshi S. (1990). Effect of Allium sativum on epididymal spermatozoa, estradiol-treated mice and general toxicity. *J Ethnopharmacol.* May;29(2):117-25.

349   Qureshi S, Shah A.H., M., Ageel T. and A.M. (1989). Studies on Herbal Aphrodisiacs Used in Arab System of Medicine. *The American Journal of Chinese Medicine.* Vol. 17, No. 01n02, pp. 57-63

350   Khodaie, L., & Sadeghpoor, O. (2015). Ginger from ancient times to the new outlook. Jundishapur journal of natural pharmaceutical products, 10(1), e18402.

351   Tajuddin, Ahmad S, Latif A, Qasmi IA. (2003). Aphrodisiac activity of 50% ethanolic extracts of Myristica fragrans Houtt. (nutmeg) and Syzygium aromaticum (L) Merr. & Perry. (clove) in male mice: a comparative study.BMC Complement Altern Med. Oct 20; 3():6.

352   Tajuddin, Ahmad S, Latif A, Qasmi IA. Aphrodisiac activity of 50% ethanolic extracts of Myristica fragrans Houtt. (nutmeg) and Syzygium aromaticum (L) Merr. & Perry. (clove) in male mice: a comparative study. BMC Complement Altern Med. 2003;3:6. Published 2003 Oct 20.

353   Banihani S. A. (2019). Testosterone in Males as Enhanced by Onion (Allium Cepa L.). *Biomolecules.* 9(2), 75.

354   Zhang Z1, Su G2, Zhou F2, Lin L2, Liu X3, Zhao M4.(2019). Alcalase-hydrolyzed oyster (Crassostrea rivularis) meat enhances antioxidant and aphrodisiac activities in normal male mice.*Food Research International.* Volume 120, June 2019, Pages 178-187

355   Gil MI, Tomás-Barberán FA, Hess-Pierce B, Holcroft DM, Kader AA. (2000). Antioxidant activity of pomegranate juice and its relationship with phenolic composition and processing. *J Agric Food Chem.* 2000 Oct;48(10):4581-9.

356   Onal, E., Yilmaz, D., Kaya, E. et al.(2016).Pomegranate juice causes a partial improvement through lowering oxidative stress for erectile dysfunction in streptozotocin-diabetic rat. Int J Impot Res 28, 234–240 (2016)

357   Wang, D., Özen, C., Abu-Reidah, I. M., Chigurupati, S., Patra, J. K., Horbanczuk, J. O., Jóźwik, A., Tzvetkov, N. T., Uhrin, P., & Atanasov, A. G. (2018). Vasculoprotective Effects of Pomegranate (Punica granatum L.). Frontiers in pharmacology, 9, 544.

358   Ammar, A.E., Esmat, A., Hassona, M.D., Tadros, M.G., Abdel-Naim, A.B. and Guns, E.S.T. (2015), The effect of pomegranate fruit extract on testosterone-induced BPH in rats. Prostate, 75: 679-692.

359   Al-Olayan, E. M., El-Khadragy, M. F., Metwally, D. M., & Abdel Moneim, A. E. (2014). Protective effects of pomegranate (Punica granatum) juice on testes against carbon tetrachloride intoxication in rats. BMC complementary and alternative medicine, 14, 164.

360   Zhang, Q., Radisavljevic, Z.M., Siroky, M.B. and Azadzoi, K.M. (2011), Dietary antioxidants improve arteriogenic erectile dysfunction. International Journal of Andrology, 34: 225-235.

361   Hosseinzadeh H, Ziaee T, Sadeghi A. (2008). The effect of saffron, Crocus sativus stigma, extract and its constituents, safranal and crocin on sexual behaviors in normal male rats. *Phytomedicine.* 2008 Jun; 15(6-7):491-5.

362   Madan CL, Kapur BM, Gupta US. (1996). Crocus sativus saffron herb and sexual effects. Saffron. *Econ Bot.* 20:377.

363   Kashani L, Raisi F, Saroukhani S, et al. (2012). Saffron for treatment of fluoxetine-induced sexual dysfunction in women: Randomized double-blind placebo-controlled study. *Hum Psychopharmacol Clin Exp.* 2012;28(1):54-60

364   Khazdair, M. R., Boskabady, M. H., Hosseini, M., Rezaee, R., & M Tsatsakis, A. (2015). The effects of Crocus sativus (saffron) and its constituents on nervous system: A review. Avicenna journal of phytomedicine, 5(5), 376–391.

365   Mollazadeh, H., Emami, S. A., & Hosseinzadeh, H. (2015). Razi's Al-Hawi and saffron (Crocus sativus): a review. Iranian journal of basic medical sciences, 18(12), 1153–1166.

366   Majid, M., Ijaz, F., Baig, M. W., Nasir, B., Khan, M. R., & Haq, I. U. (2019). Scientific Validation of Ethnomedicinal Use of Ipomoea batatas L. Lam. as Aphrodisiac and Gonadoprotective Agent against Bisphenol A Induced Testicular Toxicity in Male Sprague Dawley Rats. *BioMed research international,* 2019, 8939854.

367   Rai A, Das S, Chamallamudi MR, et al. (2018). Evaluation of the aphrodisiac potential of a chemically characterized aqueous extract of Tamarindus indica pulp. *J Ethnopharmacol.* 2018;210:118–124.

368   Homayuonfar, A., Aminsharifi, A., Salehi, A., Sahraian, A., Dehshari, S., & Bahrami, M. (2018). A Randomized Double-blind Placebo-controlled Trial to Assess the Effect of Tamarind seed in Premature Ejaculation. Advanced biomedical research, 7, 59.

369   Chaturapanich G, Chaiyakul S, Verawatnapakul V, Pholpramool C. (2008). Effects of Kaempferia parviflora extracts on reproductive parameters and spermatic blood flow in male rats. *Reproduction.* 2008 Oct; 136(4):515-22.

370   Saokaew, S., Wilairat, P., Raktanyakan, P., Dilokthornsakul, P., Dhippayom, T., Kongkaew, C., Sruamsiri, R., Chuthaputti, A., & Chaiyakunapruk, N. (2017). Clinical Effects of Krachaidum (Kaempferia parviflora): A Systematic Review. Journal of evidence-based complementary & alternative medicine, 22(3), 413–428.

371   Toda, K., Hitoe, S., Takeda, S., & Shimoda, H. (2016). Black ginger extract increases physical fitness performance and muscular endurance by improving inflammation and energy metabolism. *Heliyon,* 2(5), e00115.

372   Gupta G, Sharma RK, Dahiya R, et al. (2008). Aphrodisiac Activity of an Aqueous Extract of Wood Ear Mushroom, Auricularia polytricha (Heterobasidiomycetes), in Male Rats. *Int J Med Mushrooms.* 2018;20(1):81–88.

373   Nasimi Doost Azgomi, R., Zomorrodi, A., Nazemyieh, H., Fazljou, S., Sadeghi Bazargani, H., Nejatbakhsh, F., Moini Jazani, A., & Ahmadi AsrBadr, Y. (2018). Effects of Withania somnifera on Reproductive System: A Systematic Review of the Available Evidence. BioMed research international, 2018.

374   Dongre, S., Langade, D., & Bhattacharyya, S. (2015). Efficacy and Safety of Ashwagandha (Withania somnifera) Root Extract in Improving Sexual Function in Women: A Pilot Study. BioMed research international, 2015, 284154.

375   Sahin, K., Orhan, C., Akdemir, F., Tuzcu, M., Gencoglu, H., Sahin, N., Turk, G., Yilmaz, I., Ozercan, I. H., & Juturu, V. (2016). Comparative evaluation of the sexual functions and NF-κB and Nrf2 pathways of some aphrodisiac herbal extracts in male rats. BMC complementary and alternative medicine, 16(1), 318.

376   Lopresti, A. L., Drummond, P. D., & Smith, S. J. (2019). A Randomized, Double-Blind, Placebo-Controlled, Crossover Study Examining the Hormonal and Vitality Effects of Ashwagandha (Withania somnifera) in Aging, Overweight Males. American journal of men's health, 13(2).

377   Ambiye, V. R., Langade, D., Dongre, S., Aptikar, P., Kulkarni, M., & Dongre, A. (2013). Clinical Evaluation of the Spermatogenic Activity of the Root Extract of Ashwagandha (Withania somnifera) in Oligospermic Males: A Pilot Study. Evidence-based complementary and alternative medicine : eCAM, 2013, 571420.

378   Liang P, Li H, Peng X, Xiao J, Liu J, Ye Z. (2004).Effects of astragalus membranaceus injection on sperm abnormality in Cd-induced rats. *Zhonghua Nan Ke Xue.* 2004 Jan; 10(1):42-5, 48.

379   Hussain, S. A., Hameed, A., Nasir, F., Wu, Y., Suleria, H., & Song, Y. (2018). Evaluation of the Spermatogenic Activity of Polyherbal Formulation in Oligospermic Males. BioMed research international, 2018, 2070895.

380   West E, Krychman M. (2015). Natural Aphrodisiacs-A Review of Selected Sexual Enhancers. *Sex Med Rev.* 2015;3(4):279–288.

381   JianFeng, C., PengYing, Z., ChengWei, X., TaoTao, H., YunGui, B., & KaoShan, C. (2012). Effect of aqueous extract of Arctium lappa L. (burdock) roots on the sexual behavior of male rats. BMC complementary and alternative medicine, 12, 8.

382   MALVIYA N., JAIN S, GUPTA VB., VYAS S. (2011). RECENT STUDIES ON APHRO-DISIAC HERBS FOR THE MANAGEMENT OF MALE SEXUAL DYSFUNCTION. A REVIEW. Acta Poloniae Pharmaceutica Drug Research, Vol. 68 No. 1 pp. 3-8.

383   MALVIYA N., JAIN S, GUPTA VB., VYAS S. (2011). RECENT STUDIES ON APHRO-DISIAC HERBS FOR THE MANAGEMENT OF MALE SEXUAL DYSFUNCTION. A REVIEW. Acta Poloniae Pharmaceutica Drug Research, Vol. 68 No. 1 pp. 3-8.

384   Jiraungkoorskul, K., & Jiraungkoorskul, W. (2016). Review of Naturopathy of Medical Mushroom, Ophiocordyceps Sinensis, in Sexual Dysfunction. *Pharmacognosy reviews,* 10(19), 1–5.

385   Rossi, P., Buonocore, D., Altobelli, E., et al. (2014). Improving Training Condition Assessment in Endurance Cyclists: Effects of Ganoderma lucidum and Ophiocordyceps sinensis Dietary Supplementation. *Evidence-based complementary and alternative medicine* : eCAM, 2014, 979613.

386   Xiao HJ, Wang T, Chen J, et al. (2010). Chuanxiongzine relaxes isolated corpus cavernosum strips and raises intracavernous pressure in rabbits. Int J Impot Res 2010;22:120-6.

387   Van Gulik, R.H. (1961). *Sexual Life in Ancient China. A Preliminary Survey of Chinese Sex and Society from ca. 1500 B.C. till 1644 A.D.* Brill.

388   Kumar, S., Madaan, R., & Sharma, A. (2008). Pharmacological evaluation of Bioactive Principle of Turnera aphrodisiaca. Indian journal of pharmaceutical sciences, 70(6), 740–744.

389   Estrada-Reyes R., Ortiz-López P., Gutiérrez-Ortíz J., Martínez-Mota L.J. (2009). Turnera diffusa Wild (Turneraceae) recovers sexual behavior in sexually exhausted males.*Ethnopharmacol.* 2009 Jun 25;123(3):423-9.

390   Reyes-Becerril M., Ginera P., Jorge Silva-Jara, Macias A.,Velazquez-Carriles C., Alcaraz-Meléndez L., Angulo C. (2020). Assessment of chemical, biological and immunological properties of "Damiana de California" Turnera diffusa Willd extracts in Longfin yellow-

tail (Seriola rivoliana) leukocytes, Fish & Shellfish. *Immunology,* Volume 100, 2020, Pages 418-426,

391   Jianping Zhao, Asok K. Dasmahapatra, Shabana I. Khan, Ikhlas A. Khan, Anti-aromatase activity of the constituents from damiana (Turnera diffusa), Journal of Ethnopharmacology,Volume 120, Issue 3,2008,Pages 387-393.

392   R. Estrada-Reyes, M. Carro-Juárez, L. Martínez-Mota. (2013). Pro-sexual effects of Turnera diffusa Wild (Turneraceae) in male rats involves the nitric oxide pathway. *Journal of Ethnopharmacology.* Volume 146, Issue 1,2013. Pages 164-172,

393   Wu YN, Liao CH, Chen KC, et al. (2015). Effect of ginkgo biloba extract (EGb-761) on recovery of erectile dysfunction in bilateral cavernous nerve injury rat model. *Urology* 2015;85:1214.e7-15.

394   Nair, R., Sellaturay, S., & Sriprasad, S. (2012). The history of ginseng in the management of erectile dysfunction in ancient China (3500-2600 BCE). Indian journal of urology : *IJU : journal of the Urological Society of India,* 28(1), 15–20. https://doi.org/10.4103/0970-1591.94946

395   Chen X. (1996). Review Cardiovascular protection by ginsenosides and their nitric oxide releasing action. *Clin Exp Pharmacol Physiol.* 1996 Aug; 23(8):728-32.

396   Effects of yang-restoring herb medicines on the levels of plasma corticosterone, testosterone and triiodothyronine]. Kuang AK, Chen JL, Chen MD Zhong Xi Yi Jie He Za Zhi. 1989 Dec; 9(12):737-8, 710.

397   Gonzales GF, Córdova A, Vega K, Chung A, Villena A, Góñez C, Castillo S. (2002). Effect of Lepidium meyenii (MACA) on sexual desire and its absent relationship with serum testosterone levels in adult healthy men. *Andrologia.* 2002 Dec; 34(6):367-72.

398   Gonzales GF, Córdova A, Vega K, Chung A, Villena A, Góñez C. (2003). Effect of Lepidium meyenii (Maca), a root with aphrodisiac and fertility-enhancing properties, on serum reproductive hormone levels in adult healthy men.*J Endocrinol.* 2003 Jan; 176(1):163-8.

399   Najaf Najafi M1, Ghazanfarpour M2. (2018). Effect of phytoestrogens on sexual function in menopausal women: a systematic review and meta-analysis. *Climacteric.* 2018 Oct;21(5):437-445.

400   [1] He WJ, Fang TH, Ma X, et al. (2009). Echinacoside elicits endothelium-dependent relaxation in rat aortic rings via an NO-cGMP pathway. *Planta Med* 2009;75:1400-4.

401   Li H, He WY, Lin F, et al. (2014). Panax notoginseng saponins improve erectile function through attenuation of oxidative stress, restoration of Akt activity and protection of endothelial and smooth muscle cells in diabetic rats with erectile dysfunction. *Urol Int* 2014;93:92-9.

402   Park JY, Shin HK, Lee YJ, Choi YW, Bae SS, Kim CD. (2009). The mechanism of vasorelaxation induced by Schisandra chinensis extract in rat thoracic aorta. *J Ethnopharmacol.* 2009 Jan 12; 121(1):69-73.

403   Sandroni P. (2001).Aphrodisiacs past and present: a historical review. *Clin Auton Res.* 2001 Oct;11(5):303-7.

404   West E, Krychman M. (2015). Natural Aphrodisiacs-A Review of Selected Sexual Enhancers. *Sex Med Rev.* 2015;3(4):279–288.

405   Yang J, Wang Y, Bao Y, et al. (2008). The total flavones from Semen cuscutae reverse the reduction of testosterone level and the expression of androgen receptor gene in kidney-yang deficient mice. *J Ethnopharmacol* 2008;119:166-71.

406   Singh, S., Nair, V., & Gupta, Y. K. (2012). Evaluation of the aphrodisiac activity of Tribulus terrestris Linn. in sexually sluggish male albino rats. Journal of pharmacology & pharmacotherapeutics, 3(1), 43–47.

407 Singh S., Gupta YK. (2011). Aphrodisiac activity of Tribulus terrestris Linn. in experimental models in rats, *Journal of Men's Health*. Volume 8, Supplement 1, 2011, Pages S75-S77.

408 Haghmorad, D., Mahmoudi, M. B., Haghighi, P., Alidadiani, P., Shahvazian, E., Tavasolian, P., Hosseini, M., & Mahmoudi, M. (2019). Improvement of fertility parameters with Tribulus Terrestris and Anacyclus Pyrethrum treatment in male rats. International braz j urol : official journal of the Brazilian Society of Urology, 45(5), 1043–1054.

409 Gama, C. R., Lasmar, R., Gama, G. F., Abreu, C. S., Nunes, C. P., Geller, M., Oliveira, L., & Santos, A. (2014). Clinical Assessment of Tribulus terrestris Extract in the Treatment of Female Sexual Dysfunction. Clinical medicine insights. Women's health, 7, 45–50.

410 Akhtari, E., Raisi, F., Keshavarz, M., Hosseini, H., Sohrabvand, F., Bioos, S., Kamalinejad, M., & Ghobadi, A. (2014). Tribulus terrestris for treatment of sexual dysfunction in women: randomized double-blind placebo - controlled study. Daru : journal of Faculty of Pharmacy, Tehran University of Medical Sciences, 22(1), 40.

411 Adeniyi AA, Brindley GS, Pryor JP, Ralph DJ. (2007). Yohimbine in the treatment of orgasmic dysfunction. *Asian J Androl.* 2007 May; 9(3):403-7.

412 West E, Krychman M. (2015). Natural Aphrodisiacs-A Review of Selected Sexual Enhancers. *Sex Med Rev.* 2015;3(4):279–288.

Bonus: A Few Tips to Give You Some Game in the Bedroom

413 Frederick, D.A., John, H.K.S., Garcia, J.R. et al. (2018). Differences in Orgasm Frequency Among Gay, Lesbian, Bisexual, and Heterosexual Men and Women in a U.S. National Sample. *Arch Sex Behav* 47, 273–288.

414 Rowland D., PhD,1 Sullivan SL., Hevesi K. (2018). Orgasmic Latency and Related Parameters in Women During Partnered and Masturbatory Sex. *J Sex Med* 2018;15:1463e1471

415 Herbenick D, Fu TJ, Arter J, Sanders SA, Dodge B. (2018). Women's Experiences With Genital Touching, Sexual Pleasure, and Orgasm: Results From a U.S. Probability Sample of Women Ages 18 to 94. J Sex Marital Ther. 2018;44(2):201-212.

416 Pfaus, J. G., Quintana, G. R., Mac Cionnaith, C., & Parada, M. (2016). The whole versus the sum of some of the parts: toward resolving the apparent controversy of clitoral versus vaginal orgasms. *Socioaffective neuroscience & psychology*, 6, 32578.

417 Wallen, K., & Lloyd, E. A. (2011). Female sexual arousal: genital anatomy and orgasm in intercourse. Hormones and behavior, 59(5), 780–792.

418 Frederick DA, John HKS, Garcia JR, Lloyd EA. (2018). Differences in Orgasm Frequency Among Gay, Lesbian, Bisexual, and Heterosexual Men and Women in a U.S. National Sample. Arch Sex Behav. 2018;47(1):273-288.

419 Meston C., Hull E., Levin R., et al. (2004). Disorders of Orgasm in Women. *Journal of Sexual Medicine* 1743 6095

420 Golmakani, N., Zare, Z., Khadem, N., Shareh, H., & Shakeri, M. T. (2015). The effect of pelvic floor muscle exercises program on sexual self-efficacy in primiparous women after delivery. Iranian journal of nursing and midwifery research, 20(3), 347–353.

CPSIA information can be obtained
at www.ICGtesting.com
Printed in the USA
FSHW021629081020
74538FS